Quick Questions in
Sport-Related Concussion

Expert Advice in Sports Medicine

QUICK QUESTIONS IN SPORTS MEDICINE

SERIES

SERIES EDITOR, ERIC L. SAUERS, PhD, ATC, FNATA

Quick Questions in
Sport-Related Concussion

Expert Advice in Sports Medicine

Editor

Tamara C. Valovich McLeod, PhD, ATC, FNATA
Athletic Training Program Director
Professor of Athletic Training
John P. Wood, DO, Endowed Chair for Sports Medicine
A.T. Still University
Mesa, Arizona

Series Editor

Eric L. Sauers, PhD, ATC, FNATA
Professor and Chair
Department of Interdisciplinary Health Sciences
Arizona School of Health Sciences
A.T. Still University
Mesa, Arizona

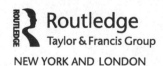

Routledge
Taylor & Francis Group

NEW YORK AND LONDON

First published in 2015 by National Athletic Trainers' Association & SLACK Incorporated

Published 2024 by Routledge
605 Third Avenue, New York, NY 10158

and by Routledge
4 Park Square, Milton Park, Abingdon, Oxon OX14 4RN

Routledge is an imprint of the Taylor & Francis Group, an informa business

Library of Congress Cataloging-in-Publication Data
Quick questions in sport-related concussion : expert advice in sports medicine / editor, Tamara C. Valovich McLeod.
    p. ; cm.
Includes bibliographical references and index.
ISBN 978-1-61711-644-5 (alk. paper)
I. Valovich McLeod, Tamara C., editor.
[DNLM: 1. Athletic Injuries--Handbooks. 2. Brain Concussion--Handbooks. WL 39]
RD97
617.1'027--dc23

2014044517

ISBN: 9781617116445 (pbk)
ISBN: 9781003526131 (ebk)

DOI: 10.4324/9781003526131

DEDICATION

To Ian, Allister, and Kalyn for your unwavering love and support.

Contents

ACKNOWLEDGMENTS

I would like to thank all of the contributing authors for their excitement about and effort toward this project and extend a special thanks to Richelle M. Williams, Lindsey Shepherd, and Michelle L. Weber for their assistance in soliciting clinical questions and editorial assistance throughout the project.

ABOUT THE EDITOR

Tamara C. Valovich McLeod, PhD, ATC, FNATA, is the Athletic Training Program Director, Professor of Athletic Training, and the John P. Wood, DO, Endowed Chair for Sports Medicine at A.T. Still University in Mesa, Arizona. Dr. McLeod completed her doctor of philosophy degree in education with an emphasis in sports medicine from the University of Virginia. She is the director of the Athletic Training Practice-Based Research Network, and her research has focused on the pediatric athlete with respect to sport-related concussion. Her current work is investigating the short- and long-term effects of pediatric sports concussion as well as recovery following concussion on traditional concussion assessments and health-related quality of life. Dr. McLeod also has research interests regarding gender differences in lower extremity function, specifically neuromuscular control and postural stability, and studies these areas through an injury prevention approach in younger athletes.

Dr. McLeod was a contributing author for the National Athletic Trainers' Association (NATA) Position Statement on the Management of Sport-Related Concussion, the lead author on the NATA Position Statement on the Prevention of Pediatric Overuse Injuries, and a consultant and contributing author on the Appropriate Medical Coverage for Secondary School-Aged Athletes. Dr. McLeod serves on numerous editorial boards, publishes frequently in athletic training and sports medicine journals, and is an NATA Fellow.

Contributing Authors

Matthew Anastasi, MD (Question 12)
Assistant Team Physician
Arizona State University
Arizona Diamondbacks and Arizona Rattlers
Phoenix, Arizona

Erica L. Beidler, MEd, ATC (Question 6)
Michigan State University
East Lansing, Michigan

Steven P. Broglio, PhD, ATC (Questions 19, 23, 25, 31)
Associate Professor
Director, NeuroSport Research Laboratory
School of Kinesiology
University of Michigan
Ann Arbor, Michigan

Javier Cárdenas, MD (Questions 26, 27)
Director, Barrow Concussion and Brain Injury Center
Director, Barrow Concussion Network
Barrow Neurological Institute
St. Joseph's Hospital and Medical Center
Phoenix, Arizona

Meeryo C. Choe, MD (Questions 20, 22)
Health Sciences Clinical Instructor
Division of Pediatric Neurology
UCLA Steve Tisch BrainSPORT Program
UCLA Mattel Children's Hospital
Los Angeles, California

Michael W. Collins, PhD (Questions 14, 18)
Director UPMC Sports Medicine Concussion Program
Associate Professor
Department of Orthopaedic Surgery
University of Pittsburgh
Pittsburgh, Pennsylvania

Tracey Covassin, PhD, ATC (Questions 6, 33)
Associate Professor
Undergraduate Athletic Training Program Director
Michigan State University
East Lansing, Michigan

Laura Decoster, ATC (Questions 2, 32)
Executive Director
New Hampshire Musculoskeletal Institute/ Safe Sports Network
Manchester, New Hampshire

R.J. Elbin, PhD (Question 18)
Assistant Professor
Director, Office for Sport Concussion Research
Department of Health, Human Performance and Recreation
University of Arkansas
Fayetteville, Arkansas

Steven Erickson, MD, FACP (Question 16)
Medical Director
Banner Concussion Center
Phoenix, Arizona

Sheri Fedor, PT, DPT (Question 14)
Outpatient Neurologic/Vestibular Program
UPMC Centers for Rehabilitation Services
Pittsburgh, Pennsylvania

Christopher C. Giza, MD (Questions 20, 22)
Professor of Pediatric Neurology and Neurosurgery
UCLA Brain Injury Research Center
Mattel Children's Hospital UCLA
David Geffen School of Medicine at UCLA
Los Angeles, California

Anthony P. Kontos, PhD (Question 18)
Assistant Research Director
UPMC Sports Medicine Concussion Program
Associate Professor
Department of Orthopaedic Surgery
University of Pittsburgh
Pittsburgh, Pennsylvania

Christina B. Kunec, PsyD (Question 14)
Neuropsychologist
Stamford Hospital Concussion Center
Orthopedic and Spine Institute
Stamford, Connecticut

Ashley C. Littleton, MA, ATC (Question 7)
Department of Allied Health Science
Interdisciplinary Curriculum in Human
    Movement Science
University of North Carolina at Chapel Hill
Matthew A. Gfeller Sport-Related Traumatic
    Brain Injury Research Center
Chapel Hill, North Carolina

*Scott C. Livingston, PhD, PT, ATC, SCS
    (Questions 5, 30)*
Program Manager, Warrior Athlete
    Reconditioning Program
Wounded Warrior Battalion East
United States Marine Corps Wounded Warrior
    Regiment
Camp Lejeune, North Carolina

Robert C. Lynall, MS, ATC (Question 35)
Doctoral Candidate
Department of Allied Health Science
Interdisciplinary Curriculum in Human
    Movement Science
University of North Carolina at Chapel Hill
Chapel Hill, North Carolina

Douglas Martini, MS (Questions 19, 23, 25)
Graduate Research Assistant
NeuroSport Research Laboratory
School of Kinesiology
University of Michigan
Ann Arbor, Michigan

Shelly Massingale, PT, MPT (Questions 16, 17)
Senior Clinical Manager
Banner Concussion Center
Phoenix, Arizona

Roger McCoy, MD (Question 12)
Head Team Physician
Arizona State University
Assistant Team Physician
Arizona Diamondbacks and Arizona Rattlers
Phoenix, Arizona

Ian A. McLeod, PA-C, ATC (Questions 4, 24)
Assistant Professor, Department of Physician
    Studies
Director of Didactic Education
A.T. Still University
Mesa, Arizona

*Jason P. Mihalik, PhD, CAT(C), ATC (Questions
    7, 11, 28, 35)*
Assistant Professor, Department of Exercise
    and Sport Science
University of North Carolina at Chapel Hill
Co-Director, Matthew A. Gfeller Sport-Related
    Traumatic Brain Injury Research Center
Chapel Hill, North Carolina

Valerie Needham, MS (Questions 34, 36)
Doctoral Candidate
American School of Professional Psychology
Argosy University
Washington, DC

John T. Parsons, PhD, ATC (Questions 9, 38)
Director, Sport Science Institute
NCAA
Indianapolis, Indiana

Danielle M.E. Ransom, PsyD (Question 37)
Postdoctoral Fellow
Division of Pediatric Neuropsychology
Children's National Health System
Rockville, Maryland

Johna K. Register-Mihalik, PhD, LAT, ATC (Questions 3, 10, 28)
Assistant Professor, Exercise and Sport Science
Research Scientist, Injury Prevention Research Center
Faculty, Matthew Gfeller Sport-Related TBI Research Center
The University of North Carolina at Chapel Hill
Chapel Hill, North Carolina

Julianne D. Schmidt, PhD, ATC (Question 11)
Assistant Professor
Department of Kinesiology
University of Georgia
Athens, Georgia

Lindsey Shepherd, MS, ATC, AT, CSCS (Question 15)
Charleston, Illinois

Amaal J. Starling, MD (Question 22)
Assistant Professor of Neurology
Division of Concussion
Division of Headache
Department of Neurology
Mayo Clinic
Phoenix, Arizona

Christopher G. Vaughan, PsyD (Questions 34, 36, 37)
Pediatric Neuropsychologist
Division of Pediatric Neuropsychology
Children's National Health System
Assistant Professor, Departments of Pediatrics & Psychiatry and Behavioral Sciences
George Washington University School of Medicine
Rockville, Maryland

Jessica Wallace, MA, ATC, AT (Question 33)
Michigan State University
East Lansing, Michigan

Michelle L. Weber, MS, AT, ATC (Questions 1, 29)
Co-Head Athletic Trainer
Desert Edge High School
Goodyear, Arizona

Richelle M. Williams, MS, ATC (Questions 8, 21, 38, 39)
Graduate Research Assistant
School of Kinesiology
University of Michigan
Ann Arbor, Michigan

Kristina Wilson, MD, MPH, CAQSM, FAAP (Question 13)
Director, Primary Care Sports Medicine
Center for Pediatric Orthopaedics, Phoenix Children's Hospital
Co-Director, Neurotrauma/Concussion Program
Barrow Neurologic Institute at Phoenix Children's Hospital
Assistant Clinical Professor, Department of Child Health
University of Arizona School of Medicine–Phoenix

Max Zeiger, BS (Question 20)
Clinic and Research Coordinator
UCLA Steve Tisch BrainSPORT Program
Division of Pediatric Neurology
UCLA Mattel Children's Hospital
Los Angeles, California

PREFACE

The Quick Questions series was developed to provide clinicians with brief, direct, actionable answers to clinical questions that they encounter in the daily practice of sports medicine to help optimize patient care. Today, information access is easier than it has ever been. However, it is a challenge to find the time and develop the skill to consume and synthesize large bodies of evidence to distill knowledge into action. Because we typically do not have the time to complete this daunting task for every clinical question that arises, we often turn to our peers and colleagues for advice. One of the most trusted sources of information in health care is the expert consult. The Quick Questions series is like having a team of sports medicine experts with you on the sidelines and in the clinic to provide you with concise, straightforward advice to answer your most important clinical questions.

The editor of each book is a leading expert in his or her area of sports medicine practice who has assembled a team of expert clinicians and scholars to develop answers to 39 of the most commonly posed and clinically important questions. Each book is a compendium of expert advice from clinicians with the knowledge and experience to help guide your clinical decision making to provide safe and effective patient care.

In this book, *Quick Questions in Sport-Related Concussion: Expert Advice in Sports Medicine*, Dr. Tamara C. Valovich McLeod and her team of expert contributing authors have answered 39 of the most important clinical questions on one of the most challenging and scrutinized areas of sports medicine. After covering some key concussion basics, this book focuses on preseason planning, assessment, management, return to play, and return to school—an all-too-often overlooked element of sports medicine concussion management.

With the busy schedules, job stresses, and time constraints inherent to sports medicine practice, it is my sincere hope that this series proves to be a valuable resource full of expert advice that you find helpful in caring for your patients and athletes.

Eric L. Sauers, PhD, ATC, FNATA
Series Editor

Introduction

Sport-related concussion is a significant issue for athletes and those engaged in physical activity at all levels of play. The issue has been given front page exposure and has led off newscasts, highlighting concussion as a mainstream media concern. The proliferation of concussion research in the scientific literature has expanded our knowledge base regarding this injury while bringing up new questions for which we may not have the answers at this point in time.

This book aims to answer many of the common questions that you may have about sport-related concussion. To compile the questions, I first reached out to colleagues working in a variety of roles and settings, including primary care, athletic training, sports medicine, neurology, and neuropsychology, and asked them about the types of questions they get asked about concussion from patients, parents, administrators, and other health care professionals. Questions were provided by athletic trainers, physicians, physician assistants, school nurses, neuropsychologists, neurologists, other health care providers, and students. The initial list of over 100 clinical questions was categorized by common themes and reduced to the 39 questions presented in the book. The contributing authors, chosen for their expertise in concussion research and/or clinical practice, were invited to write the responses for each of the questions using a mix of their clinical judgment and supporting evidence.

The questions are presented in 6 sections, beginning with issues to consider prior to a concussion being diagnosed and running through the full spectrum of postinjury assessment, management, and return to activity and school. The sections are titled (I) Concussion Basics, (II) Preseason Planning, (III) Concussion Assessment, (IV) Concussion Management Considerations, (V) Return to Activity, and (VI) Return to School. While the responses are not intended to be an in-depth analysis of the available evidence, each question and response should provide you with a quick understanding of the who, what, when, why, and how regarding many common questions about sport-related concussion.

Tamara C. Valovich McLeod, PhD, ATC, FNATA
Professor and Director, Athletic Training Program
John P. Wood, DO, Endowed Chair for Sports Medicine
Director, Athletic Training Practice-Based Research Network
A.T. Still University
Mesa, Arizona

SECTION I

CONCUSSION BASICS

WHAT IS CURRENTLY THE MOST COMMONLY ACCEPTED DEFINITION OF A SPORT-RELATED CONCUSSION, AND HOW DOES THIS DEFINITION IMPACT CLINICAL MANAGEMENT?

Michelle L. Weber, MS, AT, ATC and
Tamara C. Valovich McLeod, PhD, ATC, FNATA

Health care professionals often get asked the age-old question, "Exactly what is a concussion?" Unlike a broken bone or sprained ankle, there are no visual markers that help define the injury. Due to this, several definitions are used, and as a result, many misconceptions exist in both the medical and lay literature. Many organizations and conferences have defined concussions incorporating their own perspective. Most recently, definitions have been published by the American Medical Society for Sports Medicine (AMSSM), American Academy for Neurology (AAN), the 4th International Conference on Concussion in Sport held in Zurich, and the National Athletic Trainers Association (NATA).

The AMSSM defines a concussion as "a traumatically induced transient disturbance of brain function and is caused by a complex pathological process."[1] The statement describes concussion as a mild traumatic brain injury (mTBI) and states that all concussions are mTBIs, although not all mTBIs are concussions. Additionally, it states that concussions are a subset of mTBIs that are usually

Valovich McLeod TC, ed. *Quick Questions in Sport-Related Concussion: Expert Advice in Sports Medicine* (pp 3-6).

Figure 1-1. Traumatic brain injury spectrum.

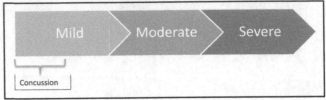

self-limited in duration and on the less severe end of the mTBI spectrum of brain injuries (Figure 1-1).

The AAN defines a concussion as "a clinical syndrome of biomechanically induced alteration of brain function, typically affecting memory and orientation, which may involve loss of consciousness."[2] This definition highlights the underlying neurometabolic cascade, cites domains that are affected, and maintains that the injury results in functional deficits rather than structural injury and that concussion can occur without loss of consciousness.

The consensus statement from the 4th International Conference on Concussion in Sport held in Zurich defines concussion as a brain injury and, more specifically, as "a complex pathophysiological process affecting the brain, induced by biomechanical forces."[3] The statement then goes on to describe many common features of a concussion (Table 1-1).[4]

Lastly, the position statement from the NATA[5] adopted the definition from the AAN with a medical panel review. This definition was adopted due to widespread use within existing literature. The position statement also recognizes the subpoints from the 4th International Conference on Concussion in Sport held in Zurich as another valid way to define concussion.

To the public, a concussion is often difficult to define. Misconceptions still exist, such as loss of consciousness being required for a concussion to be diagnosed. Others consider having a "ding" or having their "bell rung" as common and unrelated to a concussion. Research on athletes at several competitive levels has identified these misconceptions, which may lead to underreporting of concussive events. Several studies have reported that the *manner* in which concussion-related questions are asked results in different percentages of respondents who indicate sustaining a prior concussion.[6-8] Valovich McLeod et al[6] reported that approximately 8% of high school athletes identified a prior concussion history when asked using the term *concussion*; however, the percentage increased to 25% when the question was rephrased to ask about prior instances of having their *bell rung* or *being dinged*. Similarly, LaBotz et al[7] found that when concussion history questions are asked regarding whether a head injury or concussion has been sustained, 16.9% of athletes surveyed answered "yes." However, when asked if specific concussion-related symptoms have ever occurred after play, athletes answered "yes" 47.4% of the time. Other results support the notion of describing and defining a concussion based on

Table 1-1
The 4th International Conference on Concussion in Sport Held in Zurich

Common Features of a Concussion

1. Concussion may be caused either by a direct blow to the head, face, neck, or elsewhere on the body with an "impulsive" force transmitted to the head.
2. Concussion typically results in the rapid onset of short-lived impairment of neurological function that resolves spontaneously. However, in some cases, symptoms and signs may evolve over a number of minutes to hours.
3. Concussion may result in neuropathological changes, but the acute clinical symptoms largely reflect a functional disturbance rather than a structural injury, and, as such, no abnormality is seen on standard structural neuroimaging studies.
4. Concussion results in a graded set of clinical symptoms that may or may not involve loss of consciousness. Resolution of the clinical and cognitive symptoms typically follows a sequential course. However, it is important to note that in some cases symptoms may be prolonged.

Adapted from McCrory P, Meeuwisse W, Aubry M, et al. Consensus statement on concussion in sport: the 4th International Conference on Concussion in Sport Held in Zurich, November 2012. *Clin J Sport Med.* 2013;23(2):89-117.

the signs and symptoms present instead of a generalized definition. In a survey of college athletes by Kaut et al,[8] 31.9% indicated they had a previous episode where a direct blow to the head resulted in dizziness, but only 19.5% were diagnosed with a concussion. Furthermore, 28.9% reported seeing stars or colors after being hit in the head, and 26.2% indicated their head hurt at least once in the week after receiving a blow to the head.[8]

It is important as clinicians to understand the difference within these definitions, terms, and symptoms used to describe concussions when working with athletes. Athletes, parents, and coaches are not necessarily going to understand the medical definitions or the symptoms that might accompany a concussion but may describe the injury using the colloquial terms *bell rung*, *ding*, or *seeing stars*. While the use of these terms by health care providers may be warranted in getting a history from the patient, we must be careful to still acknowledge the injury as a concussion, as these lay terms may be perceived to minimize the injury or be construed as something different from a concussion. No matter which definition the clinician utilizes, it is important to recognize that a concussion is a brain injury, clinically diagnosed through the mechanism of injury and presentation of signs and symptoms. Part of our evaluation should include some education of patients and parents on the definition of concussion and the seriousness of the injury to ensure that patients and providers are on the same page while assessing and managing the injury.

References

1. Harmon KG, Drezner JA, Gammons M, et al. American Medical Society for Sports Medicine position statement: concussion in sport. *Br J Sports Med*. 2013;47(1):15-26.
2. Giza CC, Kutcher JS, Ashwal S, et al. Summary of evidence-based guideline update: evaluation and management of concussion in sports: report of the Guideline Development Subcommittee of the American Academy of Neurology. *Neurology*. 2013;80(24):2250-2257.
3. McCrory P, Meeuwisse WH, Aubry M, et al. Consensus statement on concussion in sport: the 4th International Conference on Concussion in Sport held in Zurich, November 2012. *Br J Sports Med*. 2013;47(5):250-258.
4. McCrory P, Meeuwisse W, Aubry M, et al. Consensus statement on concussion in sport: the 4th International Conference on Concussion in Sport Held in Zurich, November 2012. *Clin J Sport Med*. 2013;23(2):89-117.
5. Broglio SP, Cantu RC, Gioia GA, et al. National Athletic Trainers' Association position statement: management of sport concussion. *J Athl Train*. 2014;49(2):245-265.
6. Valovich McLeod TC, Bay RC, Heil J, McVeigh SD. Identification of sport and recreational activity concussion history through the preparticipation screening and a symptom survey in young athletes. *Clin J Sport Med*. 2008;18(3):235-240.
7. LaBotz M, Martin MR, Kimura IF, Hetzler RK, Nichols AW. A comparison of preparticipation evaluation history form and a symptom based concussion survey in the identification of previous head injury in collegiate athletes. *Clin J Sport Med*. 2005;15(2):73-78.
8. Kaut KP, DePompei R, Kerr J, Congeni J. Reports of head injury and symptom knowledge among college atheltes: implications for assessment and educational intervention. *Clin J Sports Med*. 2003;13:213-221.

HOW COMMON ARE SPORT-RELATED CONCUSSIONS?

Laura Decoster, ATC

The answer to this question is that we really don't know, and there are two main reasons for that. First, there is a limited amount of the injury surveillance data required to answer the question in younger athletes. The National Collegiate Athletic Association (NCAA) has many years' worth of data on every sport. The High School Reporting Information Online (HS RIO) project began collecting high school injury surveillance data in 2004. Data on sports injury rates and patterns in younger athletes and recreational athletes are rare. Second, the value of the surveillance data we *do* have is limited. Lack of recognition of concussion, and other impediments to reporting concussion, means it is very likely underreported. One study[1] estimated that more than 50% of concussions among high school footballers were not reported. I will present a review of the data available on the frequency of concussion. I encourage the reader to consider these data with due caution.

Valovich McLeod TC, ed. *Quick Questions in Sport-Related Concussion: Expert Advice in Sports Medicine* (pp 7-10).
© 2015 Taylor & Francis Group.

Table 2-1	
NCAA Concussions by Sport	
Sport	**Percentage of All Injuries***
Football	7.4
Men's soccer	5.5
Women's soccer	9.2
*Percentage of injuries from 2004-2009. Adapted from National Collegiate Athletic Association. www.ncaa.com.	

Exposure: How Many Could Be Injured?

The NCAA reported in 2012[2] that 453,347 athletes were participating in collegiate sports. This number is small compared with the number of children and young adults involved in recreational and interscholastic sports. According to the National Federation of High Schools, 7.7 million high school students, or more than half of all students, participate in sports. In 2012, USA Football reported that 3 million 6- to 14-year-olds play organized tackle football.[3] The National Sporting Goods Association (NSGA) annual survey for 2011[4] put the football number for all ages at 9 million. The NSGA survey also reported numbers for ice hockey (3 million), basketball (26 million), and soccer (13.9 million).

Surveillance Data: Concussion Incidence

NATIONAL COLLEGIATE ATHLETIC ASSOCIATION

As noted previously, the best data available are from the NCAA's regular surveillance efforts. In September of 2012, the NCAA reported[5] an overall injury rate of 1.9 concussions per 1000 athlete exposures (AEs) in the 16 sports they tracked. An AE is recorded anytime a student athlete steps on the field in one game or practice. In that same document, the NCAA reported the football concussion rate at 2.5 concussions per 1000 AEs. Data indicate that concussion rates have held steady over the 8 years from 2004 to 2012. Table 2-1 provides some sport-specific data.

HIGH SCHOOL

Marar et al[6] used data from the HS RIO project to analyze epidemiologic data about sports concussion in high school athletes. Published in 2012, this study evaluated concussion data from nearly 8 million AEs between 2008 and 2010. The overall concussion rate reported for the 20 sports included was 2.5 concussions per

Table 2-2
High School Concussions by Sport

Sport	Concussions per 10,000 Athlete Exposures
Football	6.4
Boys' ice hockey	5.4
Girls' soccer	3.4[a]
Girls' basketball	2.1[b]
Boys' soccer	1.9[a]
Boys' basketball	1.6[b]

Adapted from Marar M, McIlvain NM, Fields SK, Comstock RD. Epidemiology of concussions among United States high school athletes in 20 sports. *Am J Sports Med*. 2012;40(4):747-755. Boys and girls rated significantly different.
[a]*P*<.001.
[b]*P*<.03.

10,000 (ie, 0.25/1000 AEs). This is considerably lower than the NCAA rate; however, the data are not directly comparable. While the definition of AE between the NCAA and HS RIO was the same, the definition of injury for HS RIO required the injured athlete to miss at least one practice or game. There was no time-loss requirement for the NCAA definition. The Marar et al[6] study also reports that concussions represented 13.2% of all injuries that athletes suffered during the years of the study (Table 2-2).

YOUTH FOOTBALL

A recent study by Kontos et al[7] has shed some light on concussion incidence in 8- to 12-year-old football players. In this small study of youth football players from 18 teams in Pennsylvania, the incidence of concussion was found to be 1.76/1000 exposures. The authors were able to compare concussion incidence between youth aged 8 to 10 (0.93/1000 AEs) and 11 to 12 years (2.53/1000 AEs). The 11- to 12-year-old players were nearly 3 times more likely to suffer a concussion.

Centers for Disease Control and Prevention

The Centers for Disease Control and Prevention (CDC) tracks visits to emergency rooms and other health care providers in an effort to estimate the prevalence of certain conditions. A commonly cited estimate by the CDC suggests that each year there may be 300,000 sport-related concussions.[8] The October 7, 2011, Morbidity and Mortality Weekly Report[9] provides data about nonfatal traumatic brain injuries (TBIs) in sports and recreation among people 19 years and younger. Perhaps the most striking statistic in this report is that the number of emergency room visits for sports- and recreation-related concussions in young people increased 62% (from 153,375 to 248,418) between 2001 and 2009. In 2009, TBIs represented 9.4% of all nonfatal injuries seen in emergency departments for that age group. It is widely believed that this increase reflects an increase in awareness of concussion and perhaps an increase in the numbers of athletes participating in sports rather than an increase in the incidence of concussion.

Conclusion

The data available indicate that concussions are more common in competitions than in practices. Data also seem to indicate that concussions represent a considerable portion, perhaps 10% or more, of all sports injuries. Considering the millions of sports participants each year and the likelihood that concussion is underreported, calling concussion a common injury is reasonable—even if we don't know exactly how common.

References

1. McCrea M, Hammeke T, Olsen G, Leo P, Guskiewicz K. Unreported concussion in high school football players: implications for prevention. *Clin J Sport Med*. 2004;14:13-17.
2. Irick E. *NCAA Sports Sponsorship and Participation Rates Report*. Indianapolis, Indiana: The National Collegiate Athletic Association; 2012.
3. Frollo J. *Concussion education is a continuing effort for USA Football*. USA Football website. http://alpha.usafootball.com/news/featured-articles/concussion-education-continuing-effort-usa-football. Published August 8, 2012. Accessed June 4, 2013.
4. 2011 sports participation. National Sporting Goods Association website. http://www.nsga.org/files/public/2011_Participation_Ranked_by_Participation_web.pdf. Accessed June 4, 2013.
5. Hendrickson B. *Concussion rate remains steady*. The National Collegiate Athletic Association website. http://fs.ncaa.org/Docs/NCAANewsArchive/2012/september/concussion%2brate%2bremains%2bsteadydf30.html. Published September 21, 2012. Accessed June 4, 2013.
6. Marar M, McIlvain NM, Fields SK, Comstock RD. Epidemiology of concussions among United States high school athletes in 20 sports. *Am J Sports Med*. 2012;40(4):747-755.
7. Kontos AP, Elbin RJ, Fazio-Sumrock VC, et al. Incidence of sports-related concussion among youth football players aged 8-12 years. *J Pediatr*. 2013;163(3):717-720.
8. Centers for Disease Control and Prevention. Nonfatal traumatic brain injuries from sports and recreation activities: United States 2001-2005. *MMWR Morb Mortal Wkly Rep*. 2007;56(29):733-737.
9. Centers for Disease Control and Prevention. Nonfatal traumatic brain injuries related to sports and recreation activities among persons aged ≤19 years—United States, 2001-2009. *MMWR Morb Mortal Wkly Rep*. 2011;60(39):1337-1342.

WHAT ARE THE BEST EDUCATIONAL MATERIALS AVAILABLE TO HELP A COACH, PARENT, OR ATHLETE LEARN ABOUT CONCUSSIONS?

Johna K. Register-Mihalik, PhD, LAT, ATC

Educational materials regarding concussion are more readily available than ever before for clinicians, parents, coaches, athletes, and the general public. However, with so many tools and materials available, it may be difficult for clinicians to decide what may be best to use in their specific setting or with specific groups of individuals. Furthermore, the delivery method (ie, video, online, handout, interactive, lecture) of these materials and type of information presented should be considered when decisions are being made on use and implementation.

There are many educational materials and programs available, but some have more evidence supporting their use than others. The most researched of all materials is the Centers for Disease Control and Prevention's (CDC's) Heads Up program[1] (specifically the high school coaches toolkit). Other programs that are discussed empirically in the literature include the Sports Legacy Institute's Concussion Educators (SLICE) program[2] and the Athletic Concussion Training Using Interactive Video Education (ACTive) program.[3] Other videos and programming that may be useful to clinicians, but have not been empirically researched, include

Valovich McLeod TC, ed. *Quick Questions in Sport-Related Concussion: Expert Advice in Sports Medicine* (pp 11-14). © 2015 Taylor & Francis Group.

Table 3-1
Websites for Informational Materials

Material	Website
CDC Heads Up	www.cdc.gov/concussion/headsup/
SLICE program	www.sportslegacy.org/education/slice/
ACTive online program	www.brain101.orcasinc.com/1000/
National Federation for State High School Association concussion training	www.nfhslearn.com/courses/38000
National Collegiate Athletic Association and CDC concussion resources	www.cdc.gov/concussion/sports/cdc_ncaa.html
Concussion 101 YouTube links	www.youtube.com/watch?v=zCCD52Pty4A and www.youtube.com/watch?v=_55YmblG9YM
National Athletic Trainers' Association's concussion resource page	http://www.nata.org/health-issues/concussion

YouTube videos such as the Concussion 101 video and videos specific to lacrosse, football, and ice hockey developed by the National Academy of Neuropsychology (NAN) and the National Athletic Trainers' Association (NATA) in conjunction with each of the professional sporting organizations. Table 3-1 shows where these materials can be found.

- The Heads Up program materials from the CDC are free and easily accessed and include variations by sport and by audience. Specific audience versions include medical/physician practice settings, high school sports, youth sports, and school (eg, teachers and administration) information. Some research supporting the use of the CDC toolkits and resources has highlighted the ease of use and availability of the information as some of the key features of the materials.[1,4] The CDC also offers online training concerning concussion for medical professionals that can serve as a beneficial resource for expanding concussion knowledge and best practices within the medical community.

- The SLICE program, developed by the SLI's medical advisory board, is typically delivered by 2 to 3 medical professionals and incorporates PowerPoint slides, video segments, demonstrations with audience members, case studies of professional and high school athletes, personal testimonies from collegiate athletes, interactive discussions with audience members, and a question-and-answer period. The content includes signs and symptoms of concussion, long- and short-term issues associated with concussion, as well as information about responding to concussions. Age-appropriate modifications may be made for specific audiences. One published study on the SLICE program found that it was effective at immediately improving concussion knowledge among students.[2] More research is needed to understand retention. Currently, these programs are only available for scheduling through the SLI in Massachusetts, Maine, New York, and Illinois. However, there is the opportunity to start SLICE chapters in your community to deliver the program. The information is available on their website (see Table 3-1).

- The ACTive online coach, parent, and teen-athlete education program is free and available on the website (see Table 3-1). For coaches and parents, the program highlights 4 major areas: recognize, respond, return, and prevent. For teen-athletes, the 3 areas of education include recognize, report, and rest. Educator training and information are also available through this online program. Research on the coach paradigm has found significant improvements in knowledge and attitude about concussion following the program.[3]

Other specific resources that have been developed through expertise and existing evidence are available on the National Federation for State High School Association's website, the National Collegiate Athletic Association's CDC partnership website, as well as other injury-prevention organizations' websites. In addition, there are useful video tools available through various medical and sporting organizations, as well as YouTube, such as the Concussion 101 video or the National Academy of Neuropsychology/National Athletic Trainers' Association/professional sport–sponsored videos.

Most research that has been done on educational programs/materials has tested only immediate effects of such programs, so clinicians should keep in mind that a constant flow of information, or perhaps reinforcement of the information, may be beneficial in retention. Furthermore, as with any health issue, knowledge does not always equal a behavior change, so these educational programs and materials should be part of a comprehensive concussion program that creates an environment that promotes safe play and disclosure of concussion. There continues to be emerging evidence of how we can use educational tools and the effectiveness (or ineffectiveness) of these tools. Clinicians should stay abreast of this emerging evidence. In addition, clinicians should check with their state athletic associations and be familiar with their state law, if one exists, on requirements for concussion education. As clinicians work through the available materials, audience, age, sport, and resource availability should be considered to determine what materials and approaches may be best for their specific setting. In addition, the validity of the educational tools and information should be considered, as a recent study highlighted the variability in concussion educational resources that are available.[5]

References

1. Sarmiento K, Mitchko J, Klein C, Wong S. Evaluation of the Centers for Disease Control and Prevention's concussion initiative for high school coaches: "Heads up: Concussion in high school sports." *J Sch Health*. 2010,00(3):112 118.
2. Bagley AF, Daneshvar DH, Schanker BD, et al. Effectiveness of the SLICE program for youth concussion education. *Clin J Sport Med*. 2012;22(5):385-389.
3. Glang A, Koester MC, Beaver SV, Clay JE, McLaughlin KA. Online training in sports concussion for youth sports coaches. *Int J Sports Sci Coach*. 2010;5(1):1-12.
4. Sawyer RJ, Hamdallah M, White D, Pruzan M, Mitchko J, Huitric M. High school coaches' assessments, intentions to use, and use of a concussion prevention toolkit: Centers for Disease Control and Prevention's Heads Up: Concussion in High School Sports. *Health Promot Pract*. 2010;11(1):34-43.
5. Ahmed OH, Sullivan SJ, Schneiders AG, McCrory PR. Concussion information online: evaluation of information quality, content and readability of concussion-related websites. *Br J Sports Med*. 2012;46(9):675-683.

SECTION II

PRESEASON PLANNING

What Pertinent Questions Should Be Asked During a Preparticipation Physical Examination to Accurately Determine Prior Concussion History?

Ian A. McLeod, PA-C, ATC

The purpose of the preparticipation examination (PPE) as it relates to the prevention and management of concussion in athletes is to (1) establish an accurate concussion history, (2) identify risk factors and/or medical conditions that may increase an athlete's risk of sustaining a concussion, (3) identify risk factors and/or medical conditions that may predispose the athlete to concussion-related complications (ie, prolonged recovery, persistent cognitive deficits, catastrophic injury), and (4) provide an opportunity to educate and counsel an athlete and family members regarding his or her concussion risk. While the focus on this response is targeted at concussion history, it is important that clinicians understand that the medical history portion of the PPE should include a thorough neurological history and should not be solely focused on an athlete's concussion history. In order to obtain an athlete's medical history in an efficient, yet not overly cumbersome manner, screening questions are commonly utilized. It is vital that clinicians understand that the purpose of a screening question is to determine if there are areas in which the medical history should be expanded upon and examined more thoroughly. Additionally, the

Valovich McLeod TC, ed. *Quick Questions in Sport-Related Concussion: Expert Advice in Sports Medicine* (pp 17-21).
© 2015 Taylor & Francis Group.

screening questions on the PPE history form should never supplant the review of systems questions that should be incorporated into the head-to-toe examination. To maximize the history portion of the PPE, one should always inquire if the athlete completed the form or if it was completed by a family member, and in cases in which the athlete is a minor, a parent or guardian should accompany the athlete while the history portion is reviewed to ensure accuracy in the medical history.

Traditionally, the history portion of the PPE contains a battery of yes/no screening questions to identify conditions that would affect an athlete's ability to participate in sports. It has been reported in the literature that when these screening questions are utilized as part of a standardized PPE monograph, over 75% of important medical and orthopedic questions are identified.[1] The following are examples of concussion screening questions that have been commonly used in the past:

- Have you ever had a head injury or concussion?
- Have you been hit in the head and been confused or lost your memory?
- Do you have headaches with exercise?

The challenge here is that these questions are nonspecific and are dependent on an athlete's or parent's understanding of the broad spectrum of symptoms associated with concussions. As a result, the athlete's previous number of concussions may be underreported, resulting in an inadequate concussion history. A proposed solution is to incorporate questions into the PPE about the presence and frequency of concussion-related symptoms after a head injury has occurred (Table 4-1).[2,3] Including this screening method as part of the PPE has been defined in the literature as a Concussion Symptoms Survey (CSS). LaBotz et al[2] investigated the benefits of utilizing a CSS in comparison to traditional PPE questions and found that the CSS identified 71% of collegiate athletes who reported a previous history of concussion-related symptoms but did not identify a previous history of head injury/concussion. Similar results have been found in high school athletes, with 86.4% of athletes reporting symptoms on the CSS but not reporting a history of head injury/concussion.[3] The inclusion of the CSS may increase the time needed to complete the PPE, but it may improve the sensitivity and allow for more detailed information about the presence of symptoms following prior insults to the head.

Another possible solution to the problem of underreporting is to broaden the questions asked about concussion history on the PPE. This has been recommended by the International Olympic Committee in its consensus statement on periodic health evaluations of elite athletes.[4] The question included to determine prior concussion history is, "Have you ever had an injury to your face, head, skull, or brain that resulted in confusion, memory loss, or headache from a hit to your head, having your bell rung or getting dinged while participating in sports or recreational activities?"[4] This phrasing includes several concussion-related symptoms, as well

Table 4-1
Concussion Symptom Survey

When participating in athletic or recreational activities, have you ever had a head or neck injury resulting in:

Headache	No	Yes. How many times?	_____
Feeling dazed or confused	No	Yes. How many times?	_____
Dizziness or balance problems	No	Yes. How many times?	_____
Trouble concentrating	No	Yes. How many times?	_____
Ringing in the ears or sensitivity to loud noise	No	Yes. How many times?	_____
Feeling slowed down or fatigued	No	Yes. How many times?	_____
Problems with your vision	No	Yes. How many times?	_____
Feeling in a fog	No	Yes. How many times?	_____
Becoming more emotional	No	Yes. How many times?	_____
Nausea or vomiting	No	Yes. How many times?	_____
Blacking out	No	Yes. How many times?	_____
Trouble returning to activity	No	Yes. How many times?	_____
Sleep problems	No	Yes. How many times?	_____
Problem with coordination/skills	No	Yes. How many times?	_____

Adapted from LaBotz M, Martin MR, Kimura IF, Hetzler RK, Nichols AW. A comparison of preparticipation evaluation history form and a symptom based concussion survey in the identification of previous head injury in collegiate athletes. *Clin J Sport Med*. 2005;15(2):73-78; and Valovich McLeod TC, Bay RC, Heil J, McVeigh SD. Identification of sport and recreational activity concussion history through the preparticipation screening and a symptom survey in young athletes. *Clin J Sport Med*. 2008;18(3):235-240.

as the lay terminology of "ding" and "bell rung" that athletes may not necessarily identify as a possible concussion.

Regardless of the wording utilized in the initial screening questions, any athlete who indicates a "yes" response should be questioned further to determine the frequency, duration, and clinical course of the previous concussions.[1,4] Specifically, McCrory[3] suggests that follow-up questions (Table 4-2) directed at each prior concussion include the nature of the symptoms, recovery timeline, whether symptoms seem to be getting worse with each subsequent concussion, results of any diagnostic testing (eg, CT scans), and whether any head injuries resulted from non-sport participation, such as motor vehicle accidents. In addition, suspicion of concussion and the inclusion of these probing questions should be added to the PPE of athletes who sustained other injuries, such as maxofacial or ocular injuries, in which a concussion may have been overlooked.[5]

	Table 4-2
	Detailed Follow-Up Questions to Be Asked When a Previous Concussion History Is Present
Question Domain	**PPE Follow-Up Questions**
Frequency	How many previous head injuries have you had?
	Have you had any other injuries or hits to the head that you would describe as dings, bell ringers, or episodes where you felt dazed?
Mechanism	How did the injuries occur?
	Did you have any head injuries from non-sports activities such as falls or car accidents?
Symptoms	What type of symptoms did you have?
	How long did your symptoms last with each concussion?
	Did the symptoms get worse with subsequent injuries?
	Did you ever lose consciousness?
	Did you have retrograde or posttraumatic amnesia?
Management	How long were you held out of physical activity?
	Did you miss school at all?
	Did you have problems in school?
	Did your grades change at all?
Other	Is your equipment in good shape?
	Does your equipment fit well?

Adapted from Preparticipation Physical Evaluation Working Group. *Preparticipation Physical Evaluation.* 4th ed. Elk Grove Village, IL: American Academy of Pediatrics; 2010; and The International Olympic Committee (IOC) consensus statement on periodic health evaluation of elite athletes: March 2009. *J Athl Train.* 2009;44(5):538-557; and McCrory P. Participation assessment for head injury. *Clin J Sport Med.* 2004;14(3):139-144.

In addition to the specific questions about concussion, the PPE should screen for other conditions—including chronic headache disorder history (eg, migraines, tension-type headaches, cluster headaches, and medication-overuse headaches), attention deficit hyperactivity disorder (ADHD), learning disabilities, anxiety, and depression—that could possibly put an athlete at risk of prolonged recovery or confound the interpretation of postinjury symptom scores. These conditions may require modification of the concussion management plan and interpretation of neurocognitive tests and should therefore be documented on the PPE. For patients with any of these conditions, a more detailed history of their baseline symptom presentation (ie, type, frequency, severity), current treatment regime, and medication history should be obtained. Furthermore, the clinician may suggest referral for a neuropsychological consultation to establish the patient's baseline with more sensitive measures, beyond the standard computerized cognitive testing often used.

Lastly, the clinician can use the PPE as a "teachable moment" to educate the patient and his or her parent(s) about concussion, including a review of the signs and symptoms and the importance of informing a parent or medical provider if experiencing symptoms. In some cases, the PPE will identify patients who deny a concussion history, but with additional questioning (eg, CSS), it becomes apparent that they likely had a previous concussion. In addition, the clinician can use this time to discuss protective behaviors such as proper technique and avoiding aggression or high-risk situations.[4]

References

1. Preparticipation Physical Evaluation Working Group. *Preparticipation Physical Evaluation.* 4th ed. Elk Grove Village, IL: American Academy of Pediatrics; 2010.
2. LaBotz M, Martin MR, Kimura IF, Hetzler RK, Nichols AW. A comparison of preparticipation evaluation history form and a symptom based concussion survey in the identification of previous head injury in collegiate athletes. *Clin J Sport Med.* 2005;15(2):73-78.
3. Valovich McLeod TC, Bay RC, Heil J, McVeigh SD. Identification of sport and recreational activity concussion history through the preparticipation screening and a symptom survey in young athletes. *Clin J Sport Med.* 2008;18(3):235-240.
4. The International Olympic Committee (IOC) consensus statement on periodic health evaluation of elite athletes: March 2009. *J Athl Train.* 2009;44(5):538-557.
5. McCrory P. Participation assessment for head injury. *Clin J Sport Med.* 2004;14(3):139-144.

ARE THERE RISK FACTORS OR BEHAVIORS THAT CAN MAKE ATHLETES PRONE TO CONCUSSION?

Scott C. Livingston, PhD, PT, ATC, SCS

The risk of injury is inherent in sports participation, and collision sports characteristically have more acute traumatic injuries. A concussion is the most common type of acute brain injury in sports. Short-term problems associated with concussions may include increased susceptibility to subsequent concussive injury, protracted recovery, postconcussion syndrome, and second-impact syndrome. Long-term sequelae may involve mild cognitive impairment, early onset of dementia, and chronic traumatic encephalopathy.[1] The evolving knowledge and increased awareness of these short- and long-term consequences of concussions highlight the importance of minimizing initial injuries and preventing recurrent ones. Identifying and modifying such risk factors can be of significant value to the sports medicine clinician. This chapter will focus on the risk factors that can make athletes prone to concussive injuries, both initial and recurrent concussions. These risk factors include prior concussion history, sport and position played, age and sex of the athlete, genetic factors, and migraine headache history.

Valovich McLeod TC, ed. Quick Questions in Sport-Related
Concussion: Expert Advice in Sports Medicine (pp 23-27).
© 2015 Taylor & Francis Group.

Prior Concussion History

The best predictor of subsequent sport-related concussion is a history of previous injury.[1] A history of sport-related concussion is associated with an approximately 2 to 6 times higher risk of sustaining another concussion.[3,4] Among high school athletes, there is a twofold increase in concussion rate among players with a history of prior concussion, particularly among football players. Among collegiate football players with a history of 2 previous concussions, the risk for sustaining another concussion is 2.8 times greater; a history of 3 or more previous concussions increases the risk to 3.5 times more likely to sustain a repeated concussion than players with no prior concussion history.[3] Recent research also indicates that the cognitive and symptom effects of a concussion may be cumulative, especially if there is a minimal duration of time between injuries and less biomechanical force results in a subsequent concussion.

Sport, Position, and Style of Play

Certain sports, player positions, and individual playing styles have a greater risk of concussions. The concussion risk is greater for American football and Australian rugby than for any other sport. Sports with the lowest risk for concussion are baseball, softball, volleyball, and gymnastics. For female athletes, soccer has the greatest concussion risk. Although data are insufficient to characterize concussion risk by position in most major team sports, sports and player positions with frequent collisions and impacts do sustain more concussions.[5] For example, professional football backs (quarterbacks, wide receivers, running backs, and defensive backs) have 3 times greater risk of concussions than linemen[3]; kickoff plays have 4 times higher risk than rushing or passing plays. Among high school football players, linebackers on defense and running backs on offense are the most commonly concussed. Mechanisms of concussive injury vary based on sport as well as level of play.[2] The most common mechanism for concussion in athletics is player-to-player contact. In high school and collegiate soccer, for example, concussions occur most commonly from player contact and not from purposeful heading of the ball.

Position and style of play also appear to affect the risk of concussion. Improper use of the head (eg, spearing, head-to-head contact, or leading with the head), as well as improper fit of helmets or other protective equipment, may increase risk of concussion. At the high school level, over 25% of concussions are associated with illegal activity on the playing field. Aggressive behavior and violence in sports may increase concussion risk; therefore, coaches and sports organizations should address the violence and unsportsmanlike conduct that causes injury.

Age

Youth athletes are more susceptible to concussions and to concussive injuries accompanied by catastrophic injury.[2] Catastrophic injury is more likely in younger athletes and is hypothesized to be related to the physiologic differences between younger and older brains. Compared with the adult brain, the growing and developing brain of a child or adolescent may respond differently to the initial concussive impact. The developing brain differs physiologically from the adult brain based on a number of factors: brain water content, degree of myelination, blood volume, blood-brain barrier, cerebral metabolic rate of glucose, blood flow, number of synapses, and geometry and elasticity of the sutures of the skull. Any of these factors may modify the threshold to concussive injury in a child's brain. However, based on several class I studies, there is insufficient evidence to determine whether age or level of competition affects concussion risk overall because findings are not consistent across all studies or in all sports examined.[4,5]

Sex

Because of the greater number of male sports participants studied, the total number of concussions is higher for male athletes than for female athletes for all sports combined; however, the relationship between sex and concussion risk varies among sports. Female athletes are reported to have a higher rate of concussions than male athletes in similar sports. Based on class I and class II studies, it is highly probable that concussion risk is greater for female athletes participating in soccer or basketball.[5] Female athletes may experience concussive injuries more frequently due to weaker neck musculature and smaller head mass than their male counterparts. A decreased head-neck segment mass of female athletes compared with that of male athletes may contribute to greater angular acceleration of the head after a concussive impact as a mechanism for more severe injury. Male athletes may be more reluctant to report their injuries for fear of removal from competition, which may result in the incidence of concussion in boys being underestimated. Further investigation is needed to understand if sex is a risk factor for concussion and what mechanisms account for it, or if sex is merely an indicator of symptom reporting.[2]

Genetics

Genetic markers such as the apolipoprotein E4 (APOE4) gene, S-100 calcium-binding protein gene, and neuron-specific enolase have been evaluated as predisposing risk factors for concussion. Among collegiate athletes, a prior self-reported history of concussion is associated with increased odds of having either one APOE4 allele or APOE G-219T allele; in a cross-sectional study of collegiate athletes, a self-reported concussion was associated with a nearly 3 times likelihood of having APOE promoter G-219T TT genotype. However, few research studies conducted on young athletes have demonstrated significant differences in head injury characteristics or outcomes among youth athletes with these genetic markers. In a large prospective cohort study, no significant associations were observed between APOE, APOE G-219T, Tau exon 6 Hist Tyr, or Tau exon 6 Ser and concussion risk. Research studies on the association between concussions and genetic factors are limited by small sample sizes, sports populations, retrospective study design, self-reported prior concussion history (PCH), and lack of control groups. Methodological weaknesses do not support definitive conclusions on the association between genetic factors and concussion risk. Further investigation using large prospective cohort studies of representative athletic populations (controlling for athletic exposure, PCH, and other predisposing factors) is necessary to determine if genetic factors present an increased risk for concussive injuries.[2]

Migraine Headaches

A history of preexisting migraine headaches may be a risk factor for concussion and may be associated with a prolonged recovery period. An association between preexisting migraines was observed in one retrospective population study, but no association or prolonged course of recovery has been definitively demonstrated.[2] Multiple unanswered questions remain regarding a possible association between migraine headaches and concussion risk.

Conclusion

For the sports medicine clinician, implementing an effective sports concussion management program is essential to safeguard athletes and reduce long-term risks. Toward this end, 3 primary goals must be achieved: (1) safeguard the student athlete, (2) facilitate recovery and return to sport, and (3) reduce risk and liability. Researchers investigating potential risk factors for sport-related concussion (Table 5-1) have brought attention to several factors such as age, sex, and genetics, but additional investigation of these and potentially other unknown risk factors will advance our progress toward meeting these goals.

Table 5-1	
Concussion Risk Factors and Strength of Evidence	
Risk Factors for Concussion	**Strength of Evidence**
Prior concussion Participation in collision sports (men)	A: Consistent, good-quality, patient-oriented evidence
Participation in soccer (women) Female sex Age	B: Inconsistent or limited quantity, patient-oriented evidence
Migraine headache history	C: Consensus, disease-oriented, usual practice, expert opinion, or case series
Adapted from Scopaz KA, Hatzenbuehler JR. Risk modifiers for concussion and prolonged recovery. *Sports Health*. 2013;5(6):538-541.	

References

1. Sahler CS, Greenwald BD. Traumatic brain injury in sports: a review. *Rehabil Res Practice*. 2012;2012:659652.
2. Harmon KG, Drezner JA, Gamons M, et al. American Medical Society for Sports Medicine position statement: concussion in sport. *Br J Sports Med*. 2013;47:15-26.
3. Guskiewicz KM, McCrea M, Marshall SW, et al. Cumulative effects associated with recurrent concussion in collegiate football players: the NCAA Concussion Study. *JAMA*. 2003;290(19):2549-2555.
4. Guskiewicz KM, Weaver NL, Padua DA, Garrett WE Jr. Epidemiology of concussion in collegiate and high school football players. *Am J Sports Med*. 2000;28(5):643-650.
5. Giza CC, Kutcher JS, Ashwal S, et al. Summary of evidence-based guideline update: Evaluation and management of concussion in sports: report of the Guideline Development Subcommittee of the American Academy of Neurology. *Neurology*. 2013;80(24):2250-2257.

References

Are There Differences Between the Sexes Regarding Concussion Incidence, Outcomes, and Treatment?

Tracey Covassin, PhD, ATC and Erica L. Beidler, MEd, ATC

Sex Differences in Incidence

Epidemiological studies have been conducted in order to understand sex differences between female and male athletes with respect to sport injury incidence and prevalence. General trends have shown that female athletes at both the collegiate and high school levels are at a greater risk for incurring a concussion compared with male athletes in sports with similar rules and equipment. At the high school level, girls' soccer (3.6 vs 2.2 concussions per 10,000 athlete exposures [AEs] and 21.5% vs 15.1%), girls' basketball (2.1 vs 0.7 concussions per 10,000 AEs and 9.5% vs 2.81%), and girls' softball (0.7 vs 0.5 concussions per 10,000 AEs and 5.5% vs 2.9%) have higher injury rates and prevalence than boys' soccer, basketball, and baseball (Table 6-1).[1] Similarly, at the collegiate level, Hootman and colleagues[2] reported a greater prevalence of concussions in women's sports compared with men's: lacrosse (6.3% vs 5.6%), soccer (5.3% vs 3.9%), basketball (4.7% vs

Valovich McLeod TC, ed. *Quick Questions in Sport-Related Concussion: Expert Advice in Sports Medicine* (pp 29-32).
© 2015 Taylor & Francis Group.

Table 6-1

Reported Concussion Rates by Sport, Sex, and Competition Level (Rates per 10,000 AEs)

Sport	High School	College	
	Gessel et al[1] (2005-2006)	Gessel et al[1] (2005-2006)	Hootman et al[2] (1988-2004)
Football	4.7	6.1	3.7
Ice hockey (W)	—	—	9.1 [8.2]
Ice hockey (M)	—	—	4.1 [7.2]
Lacrosse (W)	—	—	2.5
Lacrosse (M)	—	—	2.6
Soccer (W)	3.6	6.3	4.1
Soccer (M)	2.2	4.9	2.8
Wrestling	1.8	4.2	2.5
Field hockey	—	—	1.8
Basketball (W)	2.1	4.3	2.2
Basketball (M)	0.7	2.7	1.6
Softball	0.7	1.9	1.4
Baseball	0.5	0.9	0.7
Volleyball	0.5	1.8	0.9

Abbreviations: AEs, athlete exposures; M, men's; W, women's.

3.2%), and softball/baseball (4.3% vs 2.5%). The data suggest that female athletes have a higher risk of incurring a concussion than male athletes.

There are several possible reasons why female athletes may be at a greater risk for sustaining a concussion than male athletes. First, female athletes tend to have weaker neck muscles and smaller neck girth, which may predispose them to an increased risk of concussion. Second, research has shown that sex differences exist in head-neck segment dynamic stabilization during head angular acceleration, resulting in acceleration/deceleration forces possibly increasing the risk for concussion. Third, female soccer athletes have a larger ball-to-head size ratio than male athletes, possibly predisposing them to concussions. Finally, research is inconclusive on whether the sex hormone estrogen leads to a greater risk of concussions.

Sex Differences in Outcomes

In addition to sex differences in the incidence of concussion, research is starting to demonstrate that female athletes may have different concussion outcomes compared with male athletes. Several researchers have suggested that female concussed athletes may take longer to recover on certain cognitive measures. Specifically, female concussed athletes have reported slower reaction time and decreased visual spatial scores than male concussed athletes. In addition to differences on cognitive measures, female concussed athletes have also self-reported more total concussion symptoms than male concussed athletes.

There are several possible reasons why female athletes may report more symptoms and have more cognitive impairments following a concussion than male athletes. Sex differences have been attributed to neuroanatomical, cerebral blood flow, and sport environment/social differences between males and females. Females have a greater area of unmyelinated neuronal processes, while males have a greater number of cortical neuronal densities. In addition, females have a higher cerebral blood flow rate than males. This increase in blood flow, coupled with a higher basal rate of glucose metabolism, may exacerbate the neurometabolic cascade. Finally, research is inconclusive regarding the potential protective or detrimental effect of estrogen on concussion outcome. Despite the growing body of research on sex differences in concussion among athletes, more research is warranted to determine clinical management of male and female athletes.

Sex Differences in Treatment

There are currently no universal recommendations for sex-specific treatments in the vast body of concussion literature. The role of sex differences in the management of concussion was debated by experts at the 4th International Conference on Concussion in Sport.[3] It was agreed that sex may be a contributing factor for injury risk and severity, but the available evidence is not yet conclusive enough to change clinical concussion management practices. As it stands, each concussive event should be managed individually with a multifaceted approach that is centered around physical and cognitive rest until acute symptom recovery occurs. Clinicians should modify concussion treatment to the specific symptoms reported by the injured person rather than the outcome differences observed between sexes in research.

Covassin and colleagues[4] proposed that sex-related differences in risk factors, clinical presentation, and management of concussions should be taken into consideration during clinical practice. Research demonstrates that females are up to 5 times more likely than males to have a personal or family history of migraine headaches.[5] This may result with headache presentation being more prevalent, severe, and longer lasting in female athletes than male athletes in postconcussion outcomes. From clinical experience, female athletes have also been reported to suffer from more anxiety issues and take relatively longer to recover than male athletes following a concussion. Due to these findings and beliefs, sport psychology and behavioral interventions may be useful to include in concussion management for female athletes in regard to their mental and physical health.

Conclusion

Researchers have suggested that male athletes have been found to be less likely to report concussive injuries to coaches and medical staff than female athletes.[3] It has also been speculated by clinicians that male athletes purposely perform worse on neurocognitive baseline tests, underreport symptoms, and attempt to present as asymptomatic in order to return to play sooner following a concussion. Clinicians should consider and anticipate these potential barriers and may need to alter their approach to concussion management for male athletes in order to protect against these problems. In order to validate and strengthen these clinical observations, further research is needed on sex-related differences in the presentation, treatment, and management of concussions.

References

1. Gessel LM, Fields SK, Collins CL, Dick RW, Comstock RD. Concussions among United States high school and collegiate athletes. *J Athl Train*. 2007;42:495-503.
2. Hootman J, Dick R, Agel J. Epidemiology of collegiate injuries for 15 sports: summary and recommendations for injury prevention initiatives. *J Athl Train*. 2007;42(2):311-319.
3. McCrory P, Meeuwisse WH, Aubry M, et al. Consensus statement on concussion in sport: the 4th International Conference on Concussion in Sport held in Zurich, November 2012. *Br J Sports Med*. 2013;47(5):250-258.
4. Covassin T, Elbin RJ, Crutcher B, Burkhart S. The management of sport-related concussion: considerations for male and female athletes. *Transl Stroke Res*. 2013;4(4):420-424.
5. Ebell MH. Diagnosis of migraine headache. *Am Fam Physician*. 2006;74(12):2087-2088.

IS IT IMPERATIVE TO PERFORM BASELINE TESTING?

Jason P. Mihalik, PhD, CAT(C), ATC and
Ashley C. Littleton, MA, ATC

Managing sport-related concussion can be challenging to many health care providers. The long-time reliance on the athlete's subjective symptom reporting is slowly being replaced by objective measures of concussion to identify cognitive, postural stability, and vestibulo-ocular deficits. In this vein, objectivity has also presented its challenges in the health care landscape.

As objective measures have proliferated the health care marketplace, it has been emphasized that these measures are best used as part of a baseline preinjury/postinjury management paradigm. It is suggested that baseline measures are collected to control for the variability in athletes' preinjury levels of cognition, postural stability, and vestibulo-ocular deficits. If an athlete later sustains a concussion, his or her baseline scores can be used as a comparison to aid in identifying postinjury deficits. Given the manner in which these tests are deployed on a wide scale, there are underlying issues surrounding the validity of baseline test scores obtained from athletes. Postinjury scores are typically captured in quiet environments and with individually motivated athletes (not distracted athletes in groups). This renders

Valovich McLeod TC, ed. *Quick Questions in Sport-Related Concussion: Expert Advice in Sports Medicine* (pp 33-37).
© 2015 Taylor & Francis Group.

comparing postinjury results to baseline results difficult and thus complicates—not facilitates—the clinical management following concussion.

What Does Reliable Change Mean, and Why Should I Care?

The premise of the preinjury/postinjury concussion management paradigm only works if an individual's performance on the tests employed demonstrates very little variability from one test session to the next. Only in this scenario can clinicians hinge on certainty that decreases in performance are likely due to the injury. This is an important aspect when considering whether baseline testing is useful. Unfortunately, the independent research on neurocognitive test platforms yields moderate-at-best reliability. One method of looking at reliability is to determine the reliable change index of a test platform's outcome measures. The reliable change index[1] demonstrates how much an individual's performance has changed, and in what direction, and whether those changes are reliable and clinically meaningful. Simply put, this method identifies the test-retest difference in scores one might expect to see in healthy individuals to place context surrounding the interpretation of any changes following injury. For example, suppose an athlete scored a 90% on the Immediate Postconcussion Assessment and Cognitive Test (ImPACT) visual memory composite score at baseline, and then scored 78% following a suspected injury (a 12-point decrease). Your immediate thought would likely be that the athlete is impaired. However, reliable change indices reveal a 14-point drop in visual memory would be necessary to signify 80% confidence that the finding is indicative of impairment.[2] Understanding these values in the context of the baseline-postinjury model is necessary to accurately interpret the results of the assessment.

Are Normative Data or Baseline Data Better?

Although preinjury/postinjury testing makes sense, the accuracy of this paradigm in the athletic realm has not been fully explored. Until randomized prospective studies have been completed, it is uncertain whether the preinjury/postinjury model possesses superior diagnostic capability over postinjury testing alone.[3] Two studies have initiated the exploration of evaluating a postinjury-only testing paradigm. In work published by our group,[4] we evaluated 258 concussed college student-athletes who completed preinjury and postinjury testing on the Automated Neuropsychological Assessment Metrics—a computerized neurocognitive test platform—and measures of balance and symptoms. We analyzed these data in 2 different ways. First, we compared each athlete's postinjury scores with his or her own preinjury scores; second, we compared each athlete's postinjury scores with normative data. For all neurocognitive measures (except for balance and symptom scores), there was no difference in diagnostic accuracy between the 2 methods. For the 2 differences, the individualized baseline comparison was favorable at identifying reaction time deficits, whereas the normative comparison was better able to identify mathematical processing deficits. Given these mixed results, and the overwhelming nondifference between both methods for all the other outcome measures, it appears that preinjury test scores—at least in an otherwise healthy sample of college athletes—may not be necessary. A clinical example demonstrating a comparison of the 2 methods is included in Table 7-1.

Echemendia and colleagues[5] also studied this phenomenon in a large sample of college student-athletes (N = 223) who had completed the ImPACT. In part, they employed only postinjury data and a criterion where athletes scoring 1.5 standard deviations below normative data were classified as injured. Their findings point to high sensitivity (ability to identify concussion when concussion exists) and specificity (ability to identify no injury when no injury has been sustained) for composite measures of verbal memory (sensitivity, 86%; specificity, 95%), visual motor speed (sensitivity, 80%; specificity, 96%), and reaction time (sensitivity, 80%; specificity, 97%). Visual memory was not evaluated in their study.

Is Baseline Testing Useful for Anyone?

It should be noted that study in this area is not yet definitive, and the results should not warrant widespread change to the preinjury/postinjury paradigms you might already have in place at this time. Normative data are usually compiled from samples of "normal" individuals. These samples usually exclude those with a pronounced history of concussion, history of attention deficit disorders or learning disabilities, or a spectrum of psychological conditions. Thus, athletes who experience these conditions would likely benefit from individualized baseline testing, provided it is carried out in a controlled environment. Younger athletes may also benefit from preinjury testing; this at-risk age group was not included in either of the aforementioned studies. As the complexity of the concussion testing marketplace evolves, subsequent and thorough study of multiple test batteries will be warranted.

Conclusion

Recent preliminary research among college student-athletes suggests that postinjury testing alone may have diagnostic value. If future research continues to support this, it will reduce the human, financial, and physical resources required

Clinical Example Comparing the Preinjury/Postinjury and Postinjury-Only Paradigms

Table 7-1

Cognitive Domain	Baseline Standard Score*	Postinjury Standard Score	RCI	Compared With Baseline: Impaired?	Normative Data	Compared With Normative Data: Impaired?
Verbal memory	124	83	20.22	Yes	90 to 109	Yes
Visual memory	107	93	17.49	No	90 to 109	No
Reaction time	95	121	9.74	No	90 to 109	No
Psychomotor speed	101	95	9.44	No	90 to 109	No

*Standard scores place all outcomes on the same scale based on age-matched normative data sets, which allows for easier clinical interpretation.

In this example, the individual was baseline tested on a computerized concussion assessment test. He later sustained a concussion and was readministered the same computerized concussion assessment test.

Preinjury/postinjury paradigm: determine if the change in scores from baseline to postinjury exceeds the RCI. For verbal memory the RCI is 20.22 and the change from baseline (124) to postinjury (83) was 41, which is greater than 20.22, indicating impairment.

Postinjury-only paradigm: baseline scores are not available; determine if the score is comparable to normative data. For verbal memory, the normative range is 90-109 and he scored an 83, which is outside the lower range of the normative range, indicating impairment.

for widespread baseline testing. Baseline testing may continue to be recommended for certain populations, such as younger athletes and those with psychiatric conditions. Clinicians should realize the limitations of objective concussion assessment tests and remember to employ a multifaceted approach when evaluating and managing concussions.

References

1. Register-Mihalik JK, Guskiewicz KM, Mihalik JP, Schmidt JD, Kerr ZY, McCrea MA. Reliable change, sensitivity, and specificity of a multidimensional concussion assessment battery: implications for caution in clinical practice. *J Head Trauma Rehabil.* 2013;28(4):274-283.
2. Iverson GL, Lovell MR, Collins MW. Interpreting change on ImPACT following sport concussion. *Clin Neuropsychol.* 2003;17(4):460-467.
3. Randolph C, McCrea M, Barr WB. Is neuropsychological testing useful in the management of sport-related concussion? *J Athl Train.* 2005;40(3):139-152.
4. Schmidt JD, Register-Mihalik JK, Mihalik JP, Kerr ZY, Guskiewicz KM. Identifying impairments after concussion: normative data versus individualized baselines. *Med Sci Sports Exerc.* 2012;44(9):1621-1628.
5. Echemendia RJ, Bruce JM, Bailey CM, Sanders JF, Arnett P, Vargas G. The utility of post-concussion neuropsychological data in identifying cognitive change following sports-related MTBI In the absence of baseline data. *Clin Neuropsychol.* 2012;26(7):1077-1091.

WHICH MEDICAL PROFESSIONALS SHOULD BE PART OF MY CONCUSSION MANAGEMENT TEAM?

Richelle M. Williams, MS, ATC and
Tamara C. Valovich McLeod, PhD, ATC, FNATA

Concussions should include a management team that encompasses a multidisciplinary approach,[1] meaning a team of health care professionals. Depending on the setting, there is a larger involvement by each medical professional; some settings only have access to a school nurse, while others have a well-rounded team of health care professionals. In all, it is important to include the following medical professionals as consultants or for direct involvement, in no particular order: athletic trainers, primary care physicians, physicians with sport medicine fellowship, school nurses, school counselors, neurologists, and neuropsychologists. These medical professionals should all be part of a concussion management team and be involved in a collaborative manner based on their specific roles, as outlined in Table 8-1. A team approach ensures that the patient receives the best care possible and enhances recovery in all aspects of impairment and throughout the recovery process. However, the responsibilities of the concussion management team may differ by state, depending on the wording of the state law pertaining to when providers are allowed to clear patients to return to activity.

Valovich McLeod TC, ed. *Quick Questions in Sport-Related
Concussion: Expert Advice in Sports Medicine* (pp 39-42).
© 2015 Taylor & Francis Group.

Table 8-1
Concussion Management Team Roles

Health Care Professional	Roles	Resource
Athletic trainer	Immediate care management/assessment	http://www.nata.org/
School nurse	Symptom assessment at school	http://www.nasn.org/
Primary care physician	Referral to further specialist Concussion management	http://www.aafp.org/home.html
Neuropsychologist	Neuropsychological evaluation Neurocognitive test interpretation	https://www.nanonline.org/Default.aspx
Neurologist	Long-term concussion management care Neurocognitive testing	https://www.aan.com/
Vestibular physical therapist	Vestibular rehabilitation therapy for treatment of dizziness, oculomotor or balance deficits	http://www.neuropt.org/special-interest-groups/vestibular-rehabilitation

Why should these medical professionals be involved with a concussion management team? All of these individual medical professionals have specific expertise and knowledge that can be vital to the recovery of a patient. Athletic trainers are typically the first to interact with a patient who has suffered a sport-related concussion. They are usually the on-site providers for sports injuries and illnesses in college and high school settings. Athletic trainers are important to the concussion management team because they have the ability to see the patient after school or throughout each day. They are able to monitor symptom improvements, relapses, and eventually return to play progressions. The athletic trainers who are familiar with and knowledgeable about proper concussion management are important and vital to returning a student-athlete back to sports and academics.

Primary care physicians can help manage concussions through prescriptions and referrals to other medical professionals. In most cases, insurance requires a patient to see his or her primary care physician prior to referral to a more specialized physician. With appropriate training, primary care physicians can help with neurocognitive testing in office and/or assist with interpretation of the neurocognitive testing results. The neurocognitive testing may be done in the athletic training room or school nurse's office, but a trained medical professional needs to evaluate and interpret the results.[2] Primary care physicians should also be involved in the initial assessment and the return-to-play decisions.

School nurses are important for facilitating follow-up evaluations during school hours in the adolescent population. In most cases, the school nurse can assist with ensuring proper care throughout the school day, including assisting with academic accommodation implementation, rest throughout the day, and monitoring of symptoms. The school nurse can facilitate a collaborative approach from after-school care to school hours and should work closely with the athletic trainer.

School counselors can assist with the implementation of academic adjustments or accommodations that may be used following a concussion. The school counselor may serve as the academic point person in the school to communicate the medical findings from the treating provider and school nurse to the teachers and other academic personnel.

A neurologist is a vital component of the concussion management team. The neurologist is especially important in long-term concussion management and can help the patient return to normal daily life. Neurologists are great consults for patients who may be in need of medications to help facilitate recovery and for patients with prolonged symptoms.

Neuropsychologists are the best medical professionals to interpret neuropsychological assessments.[2,3] In cases when further patient evaluation is necessary, neuropsychologists are the most qualified. Some patients need neuropsychological testing to better understand symptom causes, environmental factors, and any attention problems. Neuropsychologists provide a unique aspect to the concussion management team and help ensure patient recovery. Regardless of the health care provider, it is necessary to have concussion assessment training and become familiar with management protocols.

Physical therapists, especially those with specialization in vestibular therapy, are an important part of the concussion management team, especially in patients with prolonged dizziness, oculomotor impairments, or other vestibular issues. Vestibular rehabilitation therapy has been identified as a successful means to reduce dizziness and improve gaze stabilization, gait, and balance following concussion.[4]

A concussion management team helps facilitate proper recovery. Ideally, all of these medical professionals would be available for treatment and care, but not all patients have access to them. Athletic trainers, school nurses, and school counselors are not employed at every school. In some districts, the nurse and/or counselor may have responsibilities to cover several schools, which may not allow for the same level of daily involvement in the concussion management plan. It is important to receive information from well-informed and knowledgeable health care providers. As a health care provider, staying up to date with current research and literature is vital to properly treating patients who have sustained a concussion.

References

1. McCrory P, Meeuwisse WH, Aubry M, et al. Consensus statement on concussion in sport: the 4th International Conference on Concussion in Sport held in Zurich, November 2012. *Br J Sports Med*. 2013;17(5):250-258
2. Grindel SH, Lovell MR, Collins MW. The assessment of sport-related concussion: the evidence behind neuropsychological testing and management. *Clin J Sport Med*. 2001;11(3):134-143.
3. Echemendia RJ, Herring S, Bailes J. Who should conduct and interpret the neuropsychological assessment in sports-related concussion? *Br J Sports Med*. 2009;43 Suppl 1:i32-i35.
4. Alsalaheen BA, Mucha A, Morris LO, et al. Vestibular rehabilitation for dizziness and balance disorders after concussion. *J Neurol Phys Ther*. 2010;34(2):87-93.

WHAT ARE THE MOST IMPORTANT REGULATIONS AND POLICIES TO CONSIDER REGARDING THE MANAGEMENT OF SPORT-RELATED CONCUSSION?

John T. Parsons, PhD, ATC

The practicing sports medicine clinician is obligated to deliver patient care in a manner consistent with laws, standards, and scientific guidelines relevant to his or her own specialty (ie, athletic training, physical therapy). The purpose is to influence the clinician's behavior in ways that improve the quality of patient care, increase the safety of that care, or both. The clinician's failure to adhere to such policies can result in both substandard patient care and legal liability resulting from a failure to meet existing standards of care. Although sports medicine clinicians must be mindful of such policies at all times, sport-related concussion (SRC) policies are worthy of special consideration given the high level of public attention surrounding the issue and the rapidity with which SRC-related policy has emerged. Specifically, there are 4 primary sources of policies that are relevant to the management of SRC: (1) state SRC management laws, (2) state regulatory statutes and rules, (3) professional practice guidelines and position statements, and (4) standards of practice and codes of professional ethics (Table 9-1).

Valovich McLeod TC, ed. *Quick Questions in Sport-Related Concussion: Expert Advice in Sports Medicine* (pp 43-47).
© 2015 Taylor & Francis Group.

Table 9-1
Sources of Concussion Management Policy

Source	Origination	Explanation	Example
State sport-concussion management law	State legislatures	Statutes (ie, laws) establishing mandated policies and procedures for the evaluation and management of youth athletes with SRC	SB 1521 – Arizona Sport-Concussion Management Law (2011)
State regulatory statutes and rules	State legislatures; state health professions regulatory boards	Regulatory statutes establishing scopes of practice for various health professions and the interpretation of those statutes by state regulatory agencies into standing rules	ARS §32-41: Title and chapter of Arizona Revised Statutes regulating the practice of athletic training in the state of Arizona; R4-49-101 et. Seq: Arizona administrative code regulating the practice of athletic training in the state of Arizona
Professional practice guidelines and formal position statements	Member or specialty organizations; proceedings from specialty conferences; peer-reviewed publication	Condition-specific recommendations for clinical practice developed or validated by experts and based on contemporary clinical evidence	Consensus statement from the 4th International Conference on Concussion in Sport, Zurich, November 2012
Standards of practice and codes of professional ethics	Member or specialty organizations affiliated with specific health professions	Ethical or practice guidelines adopted by professional member or credentialing organizations to which credential holders and/or organizational members are obligated by virtue of their formal affiliation with the organization	Board of Certification (BOC) *Standards of Professional Practice*

The most recent examples of SRC-related policy are state sport-concussion management laws. Since 2009, 50 states and the District of Columbia have passed SRC management laws, with 36 of those statutes passed in 2011 alone. The first of these laws, and the one most responsible for shaping the form and content of subsequent laws, was House Bill 1824, known as *The Zackery Lystedt Law*, passed in the state of Washington in 2009.[1] Zackery Lystedt, a high school football player, suffered an undiagnosed concussion in a 2006 football game. Because the concussion was not identified, Zackery was allowed to return to play in the same game. A subsequent blow to his head resulted in second-impact syndrome, leaving Zackery permanently disabled.[2] The Lystedt Law established precedent for the components of sport concussion laws and was itself based on international scientific consensus about the key factors in SRC management practices.[3] While each state's bill differs to reflect local political and cultural factors, most bills establish three mandates. First, athletes and their parents must be educated about concussion and must acknowledge the risk of concussion before the athlete is allowed to participate. Second, an athlete who is *suspected* of having sustained a concussion may be removed from play or practice until he or she is evaluated by a health care professional. Third, in the event of a diagnosed concussion, the athlete may not return to participation until receiving clearance from a health care professional. These laws apply to all high school athletes, and many states have also found creative ways of extending the provisions to youth leagues when they use public school facilities.

As mentioned above, the SRC laws of each state differ, often dramatically, on these and other components. Some components, such as which health care providers are authorized to make return-to-play (RTP) decisions, can have significant impact on concussion management practices in that state. For example, Arizona has authorized 4 specific professions to make RTP decisions, including physicians (MD or DO), nurse practitioners, physician assistants, and athletic trainers. In contrast, the Lystedt Law makes only generic reference to a "licensed health care provider."[1] Consequently, a clinician unfamiliar with the provisions of a law may incorrectly assume that he or she is authorized to make RTP decisions. Complicating this situation is the fact that most state athletic associations, which govern high school sports, have passed similar but separate concussion policies that may or may not align with state concussion laws. When they do not align, providers may be uncertain about SRC management policies. For example, the Lystedt Law qualifies that the "licensed health care provider" who is authorized to make RTP decisions must be "trained in the evaluation and management of concussion," but it does not determine which Washington providers have such training. Presumably, the provider is left to determine if he or she has the requisite training before engaging in patient care. However, the Washington Interscholastic Athletic

Association has identified the specific professions it believes have the training to be compliant with the law.[4]

The second source of relevant SRC policy is the state rules and regulations that govern the practice of a health care profession within a state. Together, these rules and regulations establish a state-specific scope of practice, within which a provider must provide care in order to practice lawfully. SRC management, including RTP decisions, may or may not be part of existing state regulatory provisions for a given profession. It is also possible that while SRC management *is* a normal component of the profession's scope of practice, the sport concussion law does not specifically authorize the profession for things like RTP decision making. This situation creates regulatory ambiguity for that profession when dealing with patients subject to the jurisdiction of state concussion law, such as high school athletes with SRCs. Providers in these situations should request guidance from their state regulatory boards to ensure they do not run afoul of existing law.

A third source of relevant policy comes from consensus statements and practice guidelines published by scientific advisory councils and professional organizations. As mentioned previously, Washington's law was informed by one such document,[3] which has been updated once in the 4 years since publication.[5] These and other contemporary position statements[6,7] contribute to clinical practice guidelines—or best practices—for SRC management. Consequently, providers must remain abreast of these documents and work to incorporate their guidance into patient care practices, especially those guidelines published by the professional organizations representing the provider's profession. In other words, a practicing athletic trainer would generally be expected to practice in a manner consistent with the most recent SRC management guidelines published by the National Athletic Trainers' Association[8] because it partially establishes the standard of care to which athletic trainers will be held.

The fourth and final source of policy includes professional practice standards and codes of ethics to which health care professionals are obligated by virtue of their credentials, regulatory status (ie, licensure), or professional membership organization affiliations. These standards establish the minimal expectations for how the provider will conduct himself or herself in the course of providing clinical care. As one example, the Board of Certification's (BOC) *Standards of Professional Practice*[9] obligate athletic trainers who hold the ATC credential to practice under the direction of a physician. This is also frequently found in state regulatory statutes. The consequence of this arrangement is that athletic trainers must *always* manage SRC under the direction of a physician, which means in a manner consistent with the protocols and guidelines approved by the physician. Failure to do so could jeopardize the athletic trainer's national certification and state license.

References

1. The Zackery Lystedt Law, Engrossed House Bill 1824, Chapter 475, §2; 2009.
2. Foreman M. Sidelined for safety: new laws keep student athletes with concussions benched. *State Legislatures*. 2010;28-30.
3. McCrory P, Meeuwisse W, Johnston K, et al. Consensus statement on concussion in sport: the 3rd International Conference on Concussion in Sport held in Zurich, November 2008. *J Athl Train*. 2009;44:434-448.
4. Washington Interscholastic Activities Association. Licensed health care providers. http://www.wiaa.com/subcontent.aspx?SecID=628. Accessed September 30, 2013.
5. McCrory P, Meeuwisse WH, Aubry M, et al. Consensus statement on concussion in sport: the 4th International Conference on Concussion in Sport, Zurich, November 2012. *J Athl Train*. 2013;48:554-575.
6. American Academy of Neurology. Position statement: sports concussion. Minneapolis, MN: American Academy of Neurology; 2013:1-3.
7. Harmon KG, Drezner JA, Gammons M, et al. American Medical Society for Sports Medicine position statement: concussion in sport. *Br J Sports Med*. 2012;47:15-26.
8. Guskiewicz KM, Bruce SL, Cantu RC, et al. National Athletic Trainers' Association position statement: management of sport-related concussion. *J Athl Train*. 2004;39:280-297.
9. Certification Board. *Standards of Professional Practice*. Omaha, NE: Board of Certification for the Athletic Trainer; 2012.

References

WHAT FACTORS AID IN THE PREVENTION OF RECURRENT CONCUSSION?

Johna K. Register-Mihalik, PhD, LAT, ATC

Prevention of concussion—specifically recurrent or multiple concussions—is at the forefront of discussions in both the medical and sporting communities. There are many thoughts on efforts that could help prevent concussion, from the primary (preventing the actual event), secondary (slow or halt the disease progression), and tertiary (preventing long-term morbidities) standpoints. Primary injury-prevention measures that have been proposed for concussion involve reducing the number of head impacts an individual incurs over the course of a session, season, or even his or her career. Although few studies have elucidated the true effectiveness of such measures, a recent study in youth football highlighted that practice structure (eg, more contact practices) lead to a greater number of head impacts sustained, again providing evidence for limiting head impact exposure as an injury-prevention mechanism.[1] There are few studies like these in other sports; however, evidence does suggest that reducing the number of impacts in sports such as soccer may also have benefits.

Valovich McLeod TC, ed. *Quick Questions in Sport-Related Concussion: Expert Advice in Sports Medicine* (pp 49-52).
© 2015 Taylor & Francis Group.

Another commonly discussed primary prevention measure is using proper equipment. Although no helmet will entirely prevent concussion, having a helmet that is in good condition, worn properly, and fitted properly may reduce the chance of suffering a concussion. Studies have shown that helmets do a great job of preventing catastrophic head injuries such as skull fractures and hematomas. This is evidenced by the decrease in these types of injuries since the implementation of the modern football helmet. However, efforts are currently being made to develop helmet technology that is better at preventing concussion while still maintaining the ability to prevent the more catastrophic head injuries.

Other primary prevention efforts include proper playing technique, which ranges from heads-up hitting and tackling to playing by the rules. Head impact data show that over 20% of impacts in football still occur to the top of the head,[2] which has been shown to be a vulnerable position for head impacts and for cervical spine injury. Furthermore, good technique, field awareness, field position, and anticipation may help to mitigate head impact severity, ultimately reducing the risk of concussion.[3] Rule violations and infractions have been shown to lead to more severe head impacts than plays that follow the rules,[4] highlighting the importance of promoting fair and safe play as a preventive measure from an initial injury, as well as a recurrent injury, standpoint.

Although little research exists on their impact in reducing concussive injuries, educational programs that help athletic communities and medical providers understand how to recognize and respond to concussion when it occurs may help mitigate the sequelae of concussion. These educational initiatives should be age appropriate. Furthermore, educational initiatives should foster a playing environment that promotes safety, which includes regular discussions about concussion. In order for this to work, coaches, parents, and league administrators need to demonstrate their commitment to the promotion of safety and well-being in sport.

Most important in preventing recurrent concussion is ensuring that athletes *do not return to activity* before all signs and symptoms of concussion have resolved. Earlier research has shown that most recurrent injuries occur within the first 2 weeks following an initial concussive injury. Individuals at all levels of sport should be aware of this prevention measure and remove any athlete suspected of having a concussion from play immediately. That athlete should not be returned to play until cleared by a medical professional and until he or she is completely asymptomatic. Extra precautions should be taken with individuals with a prior history of concussion, as there is evidence to support that once an individual sustains a concussion, he or she is more likely to suffer another and to have longer recovery times.[5]

An additional strategy for secondary and tertiary prevention is having appropriate medical professionals in place to recognize, respond to, evaluate, and manage

Table 10-1

Concussion Prevention Strategies

Reduce Head-Impact Exposure

Limited contact practices

Limiting drills where contact with the head is of high risk

Proper Equipment

Properly fitted

Good condition

Properly worn

Good/Proper Playing Technique

Proper hitting/tackling technique

Correcting high-risk or bad behaviors/techniques

Fair Play

Playing by the rules

Good sportsmanship

Education and Safe Play Culture

Educational programs in place

Culture promoting disclosure and proper management of concussion

Concussion Protocol/Plan

No same-day return

Ensuring athletes do not return while symptomatic from concussion

More conservative management of athletes with prior concussion history

Comprehensive assessment and management plan in place and understood by all stakeholders

Appropriate medical coverage and access

concussive injuries that occur. Having individuals in place who can better manage these injuries creates a more positive environment for disclosure and may allow more of these injuries to be identified and properly managed, ultimately preventing some recurrent injuries and reducing the overall short- and long-term morbidities associated with injuries that do occur. Table 10-1 lists some of the most evidence-based and effective preventive measures. Overall, a comprehensive approach incorporating a combination of the strategies mentioned here will be most effective in preventing both initial and recurrent concussive injuries.

References

1. Cobb BR, Urban JE, Davenport EM, et al. Head impact exposure in youth football: elementary school ages 9-12 years and the effect of practice structure. *Ann Biomed Eng.* 2013;41(12):2463-2473.
2. Mihalik JP, Bell DR, Marshall SW, Guskiewicz KM. Measurement of head impacts in collegiate football players: an investigation of positional and event-type differences. *Neurosurgery.* 2007;61(6):1229-1235.
3. Ocwieja KE, Mihalik JP, Marshall SW, Schmidt JD, Trulock SC, Guskiewicz KM. The effect of play type and collision closing distance on head impact biomechanics. *Ann Biomed Eng.* 2012;40(1):90-96.
4. Mihalik JP, Greenwald RM, Blackburn JT, Cantu RC, Marshall SW, Guskiewicz KM. The effect of infraction type on head impact severity in youth ice hockey. *Med Sci Sports Exerc.* 2009;42(8):1431-1438.
5. Castile L, Collins CL, McIlvain NM, Comstock RD. The epidemiology of new versus recurrent sports concussions among high school athletes, 2005-2010. *Br J Sports Med.* 2012;46(8):603-610.

CAN PROTECTIVE EQUIPMENT OR STRENGTHENING THE NECK DECREASE THE RISK OF CONCUSSION?

Jason P. Mihalik, PhD, CAT(C), ATC and Julianne D. Schmidt, PhD, ATC

Very little is known about the types of forces that cause mild traumatic brain injuries (TBI) and, perhaps alarmingly, very few suggested methods to reduce head impact forces. Two ways of reducing concussion risk that are often discussed involve protective equipment (extrinsic) and neck strengthening (intrinsic).

What Is the Role of Protective Equipment in Reducing Concussion Risk?

Insofar as protective equipment is designed to protect the body from harm, existing helmet standards are established to ensure that manufactured helmets—regardless of sport or application—are capable of preventing catastrophic and potentially fatal injuries. These standards do not evaluate a helmet's capability of preventing concussion. The underlying limitation to developing adequate concussion helmet standards is that researchers do not yet fully understand the biomechanical inputs

Valovich McLeod TC, ed. *Quick Questions in Sport-Related Concussion: Expert Advice in Sports Medicine* (pp 53-57).
© 2015 Taylor & Francis Group.

that cause concussion. We remain intrigued that 2 near-identical collisions will result in injury for one athlete, while another is seemingly uninjured. Helmets that meet industry standards work well to protect athletes from catastrophic injuries and are fully capable of mitigating very high forces associated with these types of trauma. Blanket statements that helmets are fully incapable of preventing concussions should be tempered. By virtue of their capability to reduce forces transmitted to the skull and brain, they certainly help to mitigate concussion forces. They are just incapable of eliminating *all* risk of concussion. Additionally, people have looked to ancillary protective equipment to prevent sport concussions, including mouthguards and protective headbands. While spurious marketing practices may be convincing, the peer-reviewed science just does not support mouthguards or padded headbands as enabling effective concussion prevention.[1] The use of these devices *for the sole purpose of concussion prevention* should be employed with extreme caution.

Can Increasing Neck Strength Mitigate Concussion Risk?

Neck strength has long been theorized to play a role in head protection. An athlete contracting the neck musculature prior to head impact increases the effective mass to that of his or her head-neck-trunk segments combined, resulting in less acceleration of the head. When an impact is unanticipated and the neck musculature is not fully contracted, the anecdotal tenet suggests that the effective mass is reduced to approximately that of the head, rather than the head, neck, and trunk. Keeping the forces applied during a collision constant in a simple Newtonian approach (force = mass × acceleration), the head would experience substantially greater acceleration when the force acts upon the smaller effective mass of the head rather than the head, neck, and trunk segments combined. It is believed that the athlete would be more likely to sustain a concussion when the neck musculature is not tensed. Adolescent and female athletes are thought to be at greater risk of sustaining a concussion because they lack adequate neck strength compared with their adult and male counterparts, respectively.

Although this theory has existed for a long time, the potential link between concussion risk and neck strength has not been adequately studied. In one study, smaller neck anthropometrics and weaker overall neck strength were associated with an increased concussion injury risk among high school athletes.[2] Very few studies have examined the role of the neck musculature in decelerating the head following head impact, and existing studies have yielded inconclusive findings. Research that has examined the role of neck strength in reducing head acceleration among youth ice hockey[3] and football players[4] have found that players with weaker neck musculature do not sustain more severe head impacts. The neck musculature's response following head impact is not determined by muscle strength alone. In fact, athletes are not likely capable of reaching peak strength during the short time prior to and during head impact. Head protection may be a product of a player's anticipation and his or her dynamic response to the collision. Assessing neck strength alone may explain why many studies regarding neck musculature and head protection have been inconclusive. Dynamic neck musculature responses, such as muscle stiffness and muscle activation, may actually play a larger role in head impact mitigation and concussion prevention.[4] Female athletes experience greater head displacement following external load application and during soccer ball heading despite activating their neck musculature earlier and to a greater extent than male athletes, which may explain why female athletes are at greater risk of sustaining concussions.[5,6] An 8-week strength-training program resulted in neck strength increases but did not improve the dynamic response of the neck musculature, likely because the program did not include exercises aimed at improving the dynamic neuromuscular response of the neck musculature.[7] Training programs designed to enhance an athlete's ability to anticipate a collision and improve the dynamic response of the neck musculature may be a suitable and effective approach for reducing the severity of head impacts among athletes; however, more research is needed. Table 11-1 provides information related to the studies cited above.

Conclusion

Many concussion-prevention strategies have been proposed. Protective equipment and neck strength continue to gain popular strength. In light of the findings that do not support these 2 injury-prevention strategies, possible adaptations to playing style that actually increase an athlete's risk of injury must be considered. In considering these at-risk playing styles, coaches and clinicians are uniquely positioned to modify dangerous playing behaviors (eg, reducing head-down tackling). Additionally, rule changes designed to reduce injury (eg, spearing, kick-off location) may play a larger role in mitigating concussion risk among athletes.

Table 11-1

Studies Investigating the Role of Cervical Muscle Strength in Mitigating Head Acceleration and Concussion Risk

Study	Study Design	Sample Size	Sample Type	Summary of Findings
Collins et al[2]	Longitudinal cohort	2885 females 3573 males	High school soccer, basketball, and lacrosse players	Concussion risk associated with smaller neck anthropometrics and overall neck strength. For every 1 lb increased in neck strength, a 5% reduction in concussion odds.
Mihalik et al[3]	Prospective cohort	37 males	Youth ice hockey players	No difference in head acceleration between players with high, moderate, and low strength.
Schmidt et al[4]	Prospective cohort	49 males	High school and collegiate American football players	Greater cervical stiffness and less angular displacement after head perturbation reduced the odds of sustaining higher magnitude head impacts. Players with stronger and larger neck muscles do not experience less severe head impacts.
Tierney et al[5]	Cross-sectional	29 females 15 males	College-aged soccer players with at least 5 years of experience with heading	Female soccer players experienced greater head acceleration than when wearing headgear compared with males.
Tierney et al[6]	Cross-sectional	20 females 20 males	Physically active volunteers	Females exhibited greater head acceleration following load application despite greater and earlier activation of their neck musculature than males. Females also had significantly less strength, neck girth, and head mass.
Mansell et al[7]	Pre- and posttest with control group	19 females 17 males	NCAA Division I collegiate soccer players	An 8-week resistance-training program improved strength but not head-neck segment dynamic stabilization during force application.

References

1. Benson BW, Hamilton GM, Meeuwisse WH, McCrory P, Dvorak J. Is protective equipment useful in preventing concussion? A systematic review of the literature. *Br J Sports Med.* 2009;43 Suppl 1:I56-I67.
2. Collins CL, Fletcher EN, Fields SK, et al. Neck strength: a protective factor reducing risk for concussion in high school sports. *J Prim Prev.* 2014;35(5):309-319.
3. Mihalik JP, Guskiewicz KM, Marshall SW, Greenwald RM, Blackburn JT, Cantu RC. Does cervical muscle strength in youth ice hockey players affect head impact biomechanics? *Clin J Sport Med.* 2011;21(5):416-421.
4. Schmidt JD, Guskiewicz KM, Blackburn JT, Mihalik JP, Siegmund GP, Marshall SW. The influence of cervical muscle characteristics on head impact biomechanics in football. *Am J Sports Med.* 2014;42(9):2056-2066.
5. Tierney RT, Higgins M, Caswell SV, et al. Sex differences in head acceleration during heading while wearing soccer headgear. *J Athl Train.* 2008;43(6):578-584.
6. Tierney RT, Sitler MR, Swanik CB, Swanik KA, Higgins M, Torg J. Gender differences in head-neck segment dynamic stabilization during head acceleration. *Med Sci Sports Exerc.* 2005;37(2):272-279.
7. Mansell J, Tierney RT, Sitler MR, Swanik KA, Stearne D. Resistance training and head-neck segment dynamic stabilization in male and female collegiate soccer players. *J Athl Train.* 2005;40(4):310-319.

SECTION III

CONCUSSION ASSESSMENT

What Should Be Included in the On-Field or Sideline Examination to Diagnose a Suspected Concussion?

Roger McCoy, MD and Matthew Anastasi, MD

The sideline examination to diagnose a concussion is perhaps one of the most difficult tasks a sport medicine health care professional faces. Each potential concussion can be a unique clinical presentation and therefore necessitates a standard approach for initial evaluation.

Regardless of the particular sport, athletic trainers are often the first responders to any on-field injury. Before the sideline evaluation for a possible concussion can begin, an athlete's level of consciousness and cervical spine must be assessed. In addition, never forget the essential ABCs of a potential serious injury: airway, breathing, and circulation.[1] If an athlete has been deemed unconscious or if there is concern for a cervical spine injury, emergency medical services should be notified immediately.

Recognition of concussions is a very difficult assignment for a few reasons. First, the presenting complaint can consist of a broad constellation of signs and symptoms—physical, emotional, or cognitive. Furthermore, athletes often avoid sideline interaction with medical personnel when they experience concussive type symptoms because they do not want to be removed from play.[2] They may also attempt to

Valovich McLeod TC, ed. *Quick Questions in Sport-Related Concussion: Expert Advice in Sports Medicine* (pp 61-64).

minimize their symptoms. However, because of the close relationship between the athletes and athletic training staff, it may be easier to identify abnormal behaviors.

Prospectively validated signs and symptoms of concussions include amnesia, loss of consciousness, headache, dizziness, blurred vision, attention deficit, memory problems, postural instability, and nausea.[2] If any athlete experiences one or more of these symptoms, he or she should immediately be removed from competition and further evaluated. Always remove and secure the athlete's helmet before beginning your sideline assessment.

Since 2002, there have been 4 International Conferences on Concussion in Sport that have been held in Vienna, Prague, and Zurich to help guide sports medicine providers with concussion management. Throughout this time, there have been a number of concussion assessment tools that have been used on the sidelines. The last conference in 2012 produced the most current sideline evaluation tool, the Sport Concussion Assessment Tool, Third Edition (SCAT3).[3] It has been widely accepted as the best standardized tool for the sideline evaluation of suspected concussions, can be used on any athlete aged 13 years or older, and should be used in conjunction with a thorough clinical examination. However, if clinicians do not have access to the formal SCAT3, an evaluation that includes a neurological examination, balance test, and brief cognitive assessment could be used.

The goal of the athletic trainer on the sideline is to determine whether an individual sustained a concussion and to rule out more serious injury, such as an intracranial bleed. As previously stated, it is not always a simple yes or no answer. However, if you approach each possible concussion with the same systematic examination, it will become clearer with experience.

Using the SCAT3 as an outline, you can begin to question the athlete using the Maddocks Score.[4] This consists of the following 5 questions, with 1 point given for each correct score:

1. At what venue are we today?
2. Which half is it now?
3. Who scored last in this match?
4. What team did you play last week/game?
5. Did your team win the last game?

The questions for the athlete should then shift to his or her symptoms. Each symptom is graded on a scale between 0 (none) and 6 (severe). These symptoms include headache, pressure in the head, neck pain, nausea or vomiting, dizziness, blurred vision, balance problems, sensitivity to light, sensitivity to noise, feeling slowed down, feeling "in a fog," not feeling "right," difficulty concentrating, difficulty remembering, fatigue or low energy, confusion, drowsiness, trouble falling asleep, feeling more emotional, irritability, sadness, nervousness, or anxiety. All of

Table 12-1
Author's Initial Brief Sideline Assessment
Sideline Assessment Questions
What type of hit did you sustain (head to head, head to ground)?
Did you black out or see stars?
Do you have a headache, neck/back pain, numbness/tingling, visual changes?
What play was run and what was your responsibility?
Who scored last? What's the score now?

these questions should be asked during the initial sideline evaluation (Table 12-1). Regardless of the symptom score, the examination should then move to the cognitive and physical evaluations.

The cognitive assessment should begin with questions regarding orientation: what month is it, what is the date today, what is the day of the week, what year is it, and what time is it right now? The next portion of the evaluation consists of immediate memory recall and concentration questions. The athlete is given 5 simple objects to remember: elbow, apple, carpet, saddle, and bubble. He or she is asked to immediately recite them. This process is repeated three times. The concentration questioning asks the athlete to repeat 4 series of digits in reverse. The first series consists of 3 digits, followed by 4, 5, and finally 6 numbers. The concentration portion concludes with asking the athlete to state the months of the year in reverse. All of these questions are scored before moving to the physical examination (Table 12-2).

Neck examination includes testing range of motion and palpation, as well as strength and sensation of the upper extremities. In addition, you should perform the Spurling's maneuver bilaterally to assess for cervical radiculopathy. A neurological exam should also detail the preservation of cranial nerves II to XII. The physical exam should progress to Modified Balance Error Scoring System (BESS) testing.[5] This test consists of having the athlete perform a double leg stance on the sideline. The next part of BESS testing is having the athlete peform a single-leg stance using his or her nondominant leg, followed by a tandem stance with the nondominant foot in the back. All of these activities are timed, and the athlete will have his or her eyes closed and hands on hips. As the examiner, you are looking for unsteadiness, moving out of position, opening of the eyes, or movement of the hands off of the iliac crest.

The sideline evaluation should conclude with asking the athlete to repeat the 5 simple objects that he or she recited earlier for the immediate-recall portion of the examination.

By this time, the athletic trainer or evaluating clinician should have a fairly good idea of whether the athlete in question is functioning at baseline or if there is a

Table 12-2		
Physical Exam Brief Sideline Assessment		
Exam	**Findings to Look For**	**Cranial Nerves and/or Brain Components Examined**
Eye motion exam: "Follow my finger with eyes only"; plus brief visual field check	Nystagmus, difficulty tracking or focusing, accommodation causes "funny feeling," abnormal visual field	Cranial nerves: II, III, VI, VIII
Head and upper body exam	Any abnormalities with smile, opening jaw, sticking tongue out, shoulder shrug	Cranial nerves (in order): VII, V, XII, XI
Tandem Stance (BESS): nondominant foot behind dominant foot, heel to toe, eyes closed and hands on hips	Hands off iliac crest, opening eyes, step or stumble, moves hip > 30 degrees abduction, lifts forefoot or heel, remains out of test position > 5 sec	Vestibular system See SCAT3 for scoring system

noticeable deficiency on any part of his or her exam. As previously stated, the question of whether an athlete has a concussion can be a very difficult clinical scenario. However, with preseason baseline testing, a good rapport with your athletes, and a standardized approach, it becomes quite evident when someone has a concussion.

References

1. Broglio SP, Guskiewicz KM. Concussion in sports: the sideline assessment. *Sports Health*. 2009;1:361-369.
2. Goldberg LD, Dimeff RJ. Sideline management of sport-related concussions. *Sports Med Arthrosc Rev*. 2006;14:199-205.
3. Guskiewicz KM, Register-Mihalik J, McCrory P, et al. Evidence-based approach to revising the SCAT2: introducing the SCAT3. *Br J Sports Med*. 2013;47:289-293.
4. Maddocks DL, Dicker GD, Saling MM. The assessment of orientation following concussion in athletes. *Clin J Sport Med*. 1995;5:32-33.
5. Guskiewicz KM. Assessment of postural stability following sport-related concussion. *Current Sports Med Reports*. 2003;2:24-30.

WHAT ARE THE RED FLAGS DURING A SIDELINE ASSESSMENT FOR IMMEDIATE REFERRAL TO THE EMERGENCY DEPARTMENT?

Kristina Wilson, MD, MPH, CAQSM, FAAP

The most important role that a medical professional covering a sporting event plays is reducing morbidity and mortality from a secondary injury by early identification of the initial injury and appropriate management. Fortunately, the majority of sport-related injuries are injuries to the extremities. Although injuries to the head and neck in sports are not as common, they account for 70% of mortality and 20% of morbidity with permanent disability.[1] For this reason, it is important for medical professionals working with athletes to be knowledgeable about the signs and symptoms of a more severe intracranial or cervical spine injury that may be associated with the concussion. Head and neck injuries generally occur simultaneously; therefore, any suspected concussion should include suspicion of a cervical spine injury.

During the on-field assessment, the most important evaluation is to determine the extent of the initial injury and to evaluate for associated cervical spine injury or focal or posttraumatic intracranial mass lesions. Fortunately, posttraumatic intracranial injuries are infrequent but include such abnormalities as subdural

Valovich McLeod TC, ed. *Quick Questions in Sport-Related Concussion: Expert Advice in Sports Medicine* (pp 65-67).
© 2015 Taylor & Francis Group.

hematomas, epidural hematomas, cerebral contusions, intracerebral hematomas, or hemorrhages. The leading cause of death related to head injury in sport is from subdural hematomas.[1] Subdural hematomas occur when the bridging veins between the brain and dura are torn. These athletes typically present with a loss of consciousness with focal neurologic findings and may have a lucid interval similar to those athletes with epidural hematomas. Intracranial injuries often manifest over time, which is why it is critical that the athlete have serial evaluations after the injury. Reevaluation on the sideline every 5 to 7 minutes immediately after the injury provides you with the opportunity to monitor for any change in his or her exam or deterioration in his or her condition that would warrant immediate transfer to the emergency department. An associated intracranial injury should be suspected if there is a loss of consciousness, lethargy, vomiting, or change in mental status.

The decision to transport is primarily based on whether the athlete needs further evaluation with radiographic imaging due to concerns of a more extensive head or neck injury. In addition, if the athlete is unable to be monitored for deterioration in an environment with a responsible adult after sustaining a head injury, he or she should be transported for further evaluation with imaging and observation. There are several studies that have evaluated the signs and symptoms that are most predictive of an intracranial injury. These prediction rules for when to image with computed tomography (CT) scans are helpful in on-field assessments as well. These studies indicate that vomiting, physical exam signs of an underlying skull fracture, confusion (altered mental status), posttraumatic amnesia (specifically longer than 15 minutes), and loss of consciousness are most predictive of finding abnormalities with CT scan evaluation.[2] Most prediction algorithms suggest that two of these risk factors should indicate head imaging. The CT in Head Injury Patients (CHIP) prediction rule supports obtaining CT scans after minor head injury if the patient presents with vomiting, posttraumatic amnesia of 4 hours or longer, clinical signs of skull fracture, altered mental status as noted by a Glasgow Coma Score (GCS) of less than 15, or posttraumatic seizure.[3]

Head and neck injuries generally occur simultaneously. Another indication for immediate transport to and evaluation in the emergency department is concern for cervical spine injury. Cervical spine injury is often[1] associated with head injury. Annually, there are 10,000 cervical spine injuries in the United States, with 10% of these injuries being sport related. Cervical spine injury is seen in all sports, particularly diving, skiing, and surfing. Athletes can have neck pain associated with their head injury from meningeal irritation, but neck pain at time of injury should be taken seriously. Athletes with cervical spine pain should be immobilized with cervical spine precautions and transported by emergency medical services.

The last indication for immediate referral to the emergency department is signs of skull fracture. Physical exam signs concerning for skull fracture include expanding

Table 13-1	
Red Flags for Immediate Referral to Emergency Department	
Amnesia lasting longer than 15 minutes	Increase in blood pressure
Deterioration of neurological function	Unequal, dilated, or unreactive pupils
Motor deficit—weakness	Cranial nerve deficits
Sensory deficit—numbness	Vomiting
Balance deficit	Any signs of skull or neck trauma
Increasing confusion	Seizure activity
Decreasing level of consciousness	Worsening postconcussion symptoms
Difficult to arouse	Unusual personality or mood changes
Increasing lethargy	Significant irritability
Decrease or irregularity in respiration	Can't recognize people or places
Decrease or irregularity in pulse	

Adapted from Concussion: when to seek medical attention. US Centers for Disease Control and Prevention. http://www.cdc.gov/concussion/signs_symptoms.html. Published March 8, 2010..

hematoma on any area of the head other than the forehead, palpable depression, bruising behind the ears (Battle's sign, raccoon eyes), or hemotympanum. Examination of the tympanic membranes is often not performed on the sideline, but it should be if there is a high index of suspicion for an associated skull fracture.

Fortunately, most concussions are not associated with more severe intracranial injuries or cervical spine injuries. Unfortunately, these types of injuries are associated with the highest rates of morbidity and mortality in sports-related injury. Outcomes related to these injuries can be impacted by early identification and appropriate intervention with referral of these athletes for definitive diagnosis and treatment. Therefore, it is imperative that in the setting of any of the red flags in Table 13-1, suspicion of a more severe head or neck injury be raised and managed appropriately.

References

1. Ghiselli G, Schaadt G, McAllister DR. On-the-field evaluation of an athlete with a head or neck injury. *Clin Sports Med.* 2003;22:445-465.
2. Saboori M, Ahmadi J, Farajzadegam Z. Indications for brain CT scan in patients with minor head injury. *Clin Neurol Neurosurg.* 2007;109:399-405.
3. Smits M, Dippel D, Steyerberg E, et al. Predicting intracranial traumatic findings on computed tomography in patients with minor head injury: the CHIP prediction rule. *Ann Int Med.* 2007;146(6):1-55.
4. Concussion: when to seek medical attention. US Centers for Disease Control and Prevention. http://www.cdc.gov/concussion/signs_symptoms.html. Published March 8, 2010. Accessed December 3, 2014.

WHAT CONSTITUTES A "FAILED" POSTCONCUSSION TEST FOR ATHLETES WITH BASELINE NEUROCOGNITIVE OR BALANCE TESTS?

Christina B. Kunec, PsyD; Sheri Fedor, PT, DPT; and Michael W. Collins, PhD

"When it comes to concussion, don't believe me when I tell you that I'm okay." This quote from a former professional athlete exemplifies the "play through the pain" culture that is so common among athletes. Underreporting of symptoms is recognized as a frequent occurrence at all levels of competition. Athletes often fear that acknowledgement of symptoms will result in their removal from the game or even from play for the entire season. While certain athletes may purposefully minimize symptoms, others may simply lack insight into the problems and deficits they are experiencing. Recent research has shown marked memory declines lasting up to 1 week postinjury, even in mildly concussed individuals. Likewise, neurocognitive deficits have been shown to persist in athletes who report being asymptomatic at the time of evaluation.[1] Therefore, whether individuals are unaware of their deficits or simply neglecting to report them, their performance indicates they are often not fully recovered. These data have led to a reexamination of previous return-to-play guidelines that were heavily symptom based as clinicians have come to recognize the potential of exposing an athlete to additional injury.

Valovich McLeod TC, ed. *Quick Questions in Sport-Related Concussion: Expert Advice in Sports Medicine* (pp 69-72).
© 2015 Taylor & Francis Group.

More recently, neurocognitive testing has become recognized as a cornerstone of concussion management by many position papers and consensus statements. When there are concerns about the minimization of symptoms, neurocognitive testing provides objective data to assist clinicians in making decisions about the diagnosis and management of concussion. Numerous studies have shown that neurocognitive testing is sensitive to the immediate effects of concussion while not falsely identifying subtleties of normal contact in games as problematic.[2]

The number of organizations that have come to use computerized neurocognitive assessment in the management of concussion is increasing. Computerized testing is more cost- and time-efficient than having a neuropsychologist administer and interpret data for an entire team or league. This testing format also allows a large number of individuals to be tested at once with results made available immediately. Most computerized testing batteries have alternative forms that help eliminate practice effects while also providing more accurate analyses of reaction time and processing speed.

Most sports organizations require the use of baseline testing, which obtains a depiction of an athlete's neurocognitive status when he or she is presumably healthy. Baseline neurocognitive testing is particularly helpful for those individuals who have preexisting learning or attention deficits by providing a basis for self-comparison. Thus, it limits variance associated with preexisting confounding variables while detecting neurocognitive impairment and increasing diagnostic accuracy.

Concussion protocols for the majority of sports leagues emphasize "return to baseline" performance as one of the requirements to return to contact activity. When interpreting changes in cognitive performance following concussion, one must understand the probable range of measurement error surrounding test-retest difference scores. Performance on testing can be influenced by a number of factors, including repeated exposures to the test, regression to the mean, or more unpredictable forms of measurement error. Reliable change methodology is designed to identify numeric cutoffs that can be used for meaningful comparisons of test scores that are independent of practice effects and other sources of variance.[3]

When a suspected injury occurs, an athlete's postinjury scores are compared with baseline performance. If the difference between scores exceeds established reliable change cutoffs, known as reliable change indices, they are flagged as abnormal and indicative of impairment in that area. Generally speaking, a score significantly lower than an athlete's baseline performance is indicative of neurocognitive impairment in that area and precludes return to play. However, an abnormal score does not always mean "failure," and in these cases, a more thorough examination is warranted. Likewise, neurocognitive testing should always be used in conjunction with a thorough clinical interview and physical examination, which may include balance testing, before making a determination regarding a diagnosis of concussion and recommendations.

Balance testing is often used in addition to neurocognitive testing as part of a comprehensive concussion evaluation. Research has identified postural stability deficits lasting up to 3 days after injury. High-tech assessments of balance, including the Sensory Organization Test (SOT), are computerized and provide the clinician with a comprehensive report of an athlete's postural stability, sensory analysis, strategy analysis, and center of gravity alignment. Broglio et al[4] used reliable change methodology to calculate cutoff scores for each variable on the SOT, although when they were applied to postconcussion evaluations, sensitivity and specificity varied with each variable and confidence interval. These findings revealed that some concussed athletes may not exhibit large changes in postural control after injury and that this assessment should not be used in isolation to make decisions regarding concussion management.

Multiple clinical assessments of balance have been developed, including the Balance Error Scoring System (BESS), in which a trained observer assesses total errors in balance while athletes perform the tests with eyes closed on both solid and compliant surfaces. For these assessments, athletes are scored on balance errors, with more errors indicating worse postural stability control. Exertion, fatigue, and busy environments can negatively impact performance, as well as history of ankle instability. Certain researchers suggest that postural stability measures should be used only in the first few days after a concussion. Additionally, performance on assessments such as the BESS can show practice effects when administered over brief retest intervals.[5] For both computerized and clinical balance assessments, normative data exist; however, there is limited research identifying strict cutoffs for determining meaningful change from baseline. Further, these assessments only assess the vestibulospinal aspect of the vestibular system when, in fact, there may be vestibulo-ocular and ocular motor impairments as well.

Neurocognitive and balance testing are meant only to supplement—not replace—clinical judgment. Furthermore, the use of baseline assessments is meant to assist clinicians in identifying impairments after injury, not whether an individual has passed or failed the test. The determination of deterioration and then subsequent improvement in functioning and recovery following concussion is a complex clinical process that involves numerous sources of data. Thus, interpretation of these results should be left up to professionals who are trained in the assessment and management of concussion. Neuropsychologists, by virtue of background and training, are identified as being the most competent in interpreting cognitive testing results, whereas those with training in balance assessment scoring and interpretation should evaluate those test results.

References

1. Van Kampen DA, Lovell MR, Pardini JE, Collins MW, Fu F. The "value added" of neurocognitive testing after sports-related concussion. *Am J Sports Med*. 2006;34(10):1630-1635.
2. Miller JR, Adamson GJ, Pink MM, Sweet JC. Comparison of preseason, midseason, and postseason neurocognitive scores in uninjured collegiate football players. *Am J Sports Med*. 2007;35(8):1284-1288.
3. Iverson GL, Lovell MR, Collins MW. Interpreting change on ImPACT following sport concussion. *Clin Neuropsychol*. 2003;17(4):460-467.
4. Broglio SP, Ferrara MS, Sopiarz K, Kelly MS. Reliable change of the sensory organization test. *Clin J Sports Med*. 2008;18(2):148-154.
5. Iverson GL, Kaarto ML, Koehle MS. Normative data for the balance error scoring system: implications for brain injury evaluations. *Brain Injury*. 2008;22(2):147-152.

WHICH SELF-REPORT SYMPTOM SCALES ARE THE BEST FOR CONCUSSION ASSESSMENT?

Lindsey Shepherd, MS, ATC, AT, CSCS and
Tamara C. Valovich McLeod, PhD, ATC, FNATA

Medical providers often rely on symptoms reported by the athlete and the signs noticed by the clinician to come to a diagnosis of concussion. There are many different symptom scales or checklists that can be utilized to rate the type, number, severity, or duration of symptoms reported by the patient. Often, the terms *checklist* and *scale* are interchangeable in clinical practice and in the published literature. However, scales are most often graded on a 0-to-6 Likert scale, with 0 indicating the symptom is absent, 1 to 2 mild, 3 to 4 moderate, 5 to 6 severe,[1,2] whereas a checklist is often answered with a yes or no. In addition to the type of scale or checklist used, the mode of administration is also important. The scale/checklist may be verbally administered by the medical provider, or patients may be asked to self-rate their symptoms on paper or as part of a computerized neurocognitive test. Wording on the scales/checklists generally utilizes language that is easily understandable to avoid ambiguity[1]; however, clinicians need to be aware that the symptom presentation must be age appropriate.[3]

Valovich McLeod TC, ed. *Quick Questions in Sport-Related
Concussion: Expert Advice in Sports Medicine* (pp 73-78).
© 2015 Taylor & Francis Group.

There are numerous scales and checklists available for the evaluation of concussion-related symptoms. This chapter will focus on 4 scales/checklists that are commonly used in practice today. We are choosing these 4 because they can be easily accessed by providers, they are supported by research, the instructions and symptoms are easily understandable, and they have been reliable in both the adult and pediatric populations.[1,2] Table 15-1 lists the symptoms recorded on each of these 4 scales in the physical/somatic, cognitive, emotional-affective, and sleep domains.

Graded Symptom Checklist

The graded symptom checklist (GSC) is a checklist of 17 to 20 symptoms.[1] The GSC is a document that is administered to an athlete at baseline testing and again after sustaining a concussion to assist with the identification of symptoms the patient is experiencing. In addition, the GSC also pinpoints to what extent the severity of the symptoms are affecting the athlete (0-to-6 Likert scale). From the GSC, one can calculate a total symptom score (TSS) and total symptom endorsed (TSE). TSS is computed by summing the total number of symptoms out of a maximum possible. TSE reflects the total number of symptoms the athlete rates at 1 or higher. TSE allows the provider a picture of how many total symptoms the patient is experiencing as a result of the concussion. The GSC has been found to be reliable and valid.[1,4]

Postconcussion Scale

The Postconcussion Scale (PCS) is one of the oldest scales used, as well as one of the most widely used, because it has been embedded into several neurocognitive exams.[5] The PCS has 22 symptoms that are rated in severity from 0 to 6 on a Likert scale. The scale asks athletes how they feel the day the scale is given. The PCS was developed to give clinicians an objective measure on athletes' symptoms that are subjective in nature in the acute phases of concussion management.[5] The PCS has been found to be consistently reliable and valid.[3]

Acute Concussion Evaluation

The Acute Concussion Evaluation (ACE) document is a more thorough evaluation form that includes a symptom checklist. The ACE comprises a list of 26 symptoms that are self-reported by the athlete in a yes/no response format. The form also provides space for the provider to document injury characteristics.[3] This form also serves as an education resource for parents with a section on concussion

Table 15-1

Symptoms Present on Each Scale or Checklist

Symptom	GSC	PCS	ACE	SCAT3
Physical/Somatic				
Headache	X	X	X	X
Pressure in head				X
Neck pain				X
Nausea	X	X	X	X
Vomiting		X	X	X
Dizziness	X	X	X	X
Blurred vision	X	X	X	X
Vacant stare/glossy eyed	X			
Seeing stars	X			
Balance problems	X	X	X	X
Sensitivity to light	X	X	X	X
Sensitivity to noise	X	X	X	X
Ringing in the ears	X			
Numbness or tingling		X	X	
Cognitive				
Feeling slowed down	X	X	X	X
Feeling "in a fog"	X	X	X	X
Not feeling "right"				X
Difficulty concentrating	X	X	X	X
Difficulty remembering	X	X	X	X
Confusion				X
Easily distracted	X			
Loss of orientation	X			
Sleep-Related				
Fatigue or low energy	X	X	X	X
Drowsiness	X	X	X	X
Trouble falling asleep		X	X	X
Sleeping less		X	X	
Sleeping more than usual	X	X	X	
Sleep disturbance	X			

(continued)

Table 15-1 (continued) **Symptoms Present on Each Scale or Checklist**				
Symptom	GSC	PCS	ACE	SCAT3
Emotional-Affective				
More emotional	X	X	X	X
Irritability	X	X	X	X
Sadness	X	X	X	X
Nervousness/anxious	X	X	X	X
Personality change	X			
Abbreviations: ACE, Acute Concussion Scale; GSC, Graded Symptom Scale; PCS, Postconcussion Scale; SCAT3, Sport Concussion Assessment Tool, 3rd Edition.				

red flags, which indicate when to pursue further medical care at the emergency room. The ACE also contains additional information for parents on symptoms that may indicate a more prolonged recovery, as well as instructions for any follow-ups.[2] The ACE document can easily be used within the school system, allowing other health care providers to provide care when the athletic trainer is not present. The ACE document also outlines the return-to-play progression and highlights areas of which parents need to be aware as their child returns to the classroom.

Sport Concussion Assessment Tool, 3rd Edition

The Sport Concussion Assessment Tool (SCAT) was proposed in 2004 by the International Concussion in Sport group. The SCAT is a comprehensive screening concussion document that includes a symptom checklist, cognitive test, and balance assessment. The symptom scale consists of 22 concussion symptoms identified in the SCAT document, which was developed by concussion experts with the best available information at the time.[1] Over the years, the SCAT has been revised and updated based on current research. Since its inception, there have been 2 updates: the SCAT2 in 2008 and the SCAT3 in 2012. The 22 symptoms are once again rated on the standard 6-point Likert scale. The SCAT and its revisions utilize different symptoms than those generally embedded within neurocognitive tests. In 2012, the committee developed a SCAT3 for children. The Child SCAT uses different wording that is considered more age and reading level appropriate for those aged 5 to 12 years. The child version also allows parents to identify areas in which they see their child struggling, thus providing valuable insight to the health care provider. The SCAT has been found valid and reliable in published work and is also agreed upon by concussion experts.[1,5]

When deciding which symptom tool is best for an individual situation, keep in mind the age of the patient and the availability of the tool. The GSC and ACE tools have been studied in children under 12 years.[3] The GSC, ACE, and PCS have been widely studied on the high school age and older populations.[3] However, the terms used on these scales may not be appropriate for children under the age of 10 years.

Another important factor is determining when and how the checklist will be administered. Will it be by interview, or will the clinician hand a checklist to the patient? Will the checklist be administered through the computer, as is often the case during baseline administration of computerized neurocognitive tests? The provider needs to be aware that there is a benefit to interviewing patients because they are more likely to give an honest answer rather than just scoring every symptom a zero. As for a baseline test, the test administrator needs to reiterate the importance of reading directions in order to have an accurate description of the symptom reports.

The day of injury may require multiple administrations—one close to the time of injury and a second after a period of time to determine if symptoms are beginning to resolve or are becoming worse—as a means to identify red flags for immediate referral to the emergency department. In the days following the injury, it is advised that the scale or checklist be administered at least once every 24 hours. It may also be beneficial for a school nurse to administer the scale/checklist at the beginning of the day and then administer it again at the end of the day to monitor how school is affecting the individual's symptom report. It is also recommended that the scale or checklist be given before beginning each return-to-play progression step, as well as administration *after* completing the progression step to evaluate how physical activity changed symptom reports. The presence of symptoms will help guide further progression.

Conclusion

Symptom checklists and scales are important tools in helping medical professionals evaluate and manage a concussion. Selecting the appropriate symptom scale or checklist will help ensure the patient receives the best care and is returned to competition in an effective and safe manner.

References

1. Alla S, Sullivan SJ, Hale L, McCrory P. Self-report scales/checklists for the measurement of concussion symptoms: a systematic review. *Br J Sports Med*. 2009;43:(Suppl I):i3-i12.

2. Gioia GA, Collins M, Isquith PK. Improving diagnosis and identification of mild traumatic brain injury with evidence: psychometric support for the acute concussion evaluation. *J Head Trauma Rahabil.* 2008;23:230-242.

3. Gioia GA, Schneider JC, Vaughan CG, Isquith PK. Which symptom assessments and approaches are uniquely appropriate for paediatric concussion? *Br J Sports Med.* 2009;43:(Suppl I):i13–i22.

4. Piland SG, Motl RW, Guskiewicz KM, McCrea M, Ferrara MS. Structural validity of a self-report concussion-related symptom scale. *Med Sci Sports Exerc.* 2006;38:27-32.

5. Lovell MR, Iverson GL, Collins MW, et al. Measurement of symptoms following sports-related concussion: reliability and normative data for the post-concussion scale. *Appl Neuropsychol.* 2006;13:166-174.

ARE OCULAR MOVEMENTS RELATED TO CONCUSSION ASSESSMENT, AND IF SO, HOW DO I MEASURE THIS?

Steven Erickson, MD, FACP and Shelly Massingale, PT, MPT

Symptoms of dizziness and visual problems following a concussion are among the most common symptoms reported and are catching the attention of the medical community. Recent advances in the understanding of how the brain processes visual information and how it integrates with the central and peripheral vestibular system is helping to advance the examination and treatment of athletes who suffer a concussion.[1] Vision and ocular movements should always be included in the assessment and treatment of concussions. The assessment of the ocular movements should be included in any concussion evaluation as part of your clinical exam and cranial nerve assessment, and it can be done in an office setting or during a sideline assessment of concussion (Table 16-1). If there appears to be a greater need for a more in-depth evaluation, referral to a neuro-optometrist is recommended.

Valovich McLeod TC, ed. *Quick Questions in Sport-Related Concussion: Expert Advice in Sports Medicine* (pp 79-83). © 2015 Taylor & Francis Group.

Table 16-1

Assessments in an Oculomotor Examination

Ocular Movement	Evaluation Test	Clinician Assessment	Common Symptoms	Positive Test Results
Smooth pursuits	H-pattern assessment and circular pattern assessment	Quality and speed of eye movement	Double vision, headache, dizziness, difficulty focusing	Nystagmus or jumping of the eyes, difficulty following objects
Pupillary assessment	Hippus response test	Constriction of pupil with direct light	Sensitivity to light, headache	Pupil will constrict then expand while light is directed in the eye
Saccaddes	Horizontal and vertical saccade testing	Quality and speed of saccadic eye movement	Difficulty with moving eyes rapidly from one target to the next, dizziness, headache, blurred vision	Eyes do not move quickly from one object to the next, nystagmus or jumping as the eyes move, sluggishness of movement
Convergence insufficiency	Near point of convergence	Convergence of eyes when focus stick is brought up to the nose	Headache, difficulty focusing, pressure behind eyes	Double vision of the focus stick at distances greater than 10 cm
Vestibulo-ocular reflex	VOR testing or head thrust test	Passive head movement while eyes remained focused on stationary object	Headaches, dizziness, nausea, difficulty focusing	Eyes do not remain focused on stationary target and jump from side to side or up and down while head is moving

Smooth Pursuits

In evaluating the eyes following traumatic brain injury (TBI), it is important to have a systematic approach and attention to detail. Most providers assess extraocular muscles utilizing an H pattern of motion. In this testing of smooth pursuits, the provider can document adequately if all of the extraocular muscle movements are intact. When evaluating an athlete who has a third cranial nerve palsy, the affected eye cannot move medially from the midline and typically points laterally with central gaze. With fourth cranial nerve palsies, the affected eye cannot turn inward and down, and with injury to the sixth cranial nerve, the affected eye cannot fully turn outward. Each of these abnormalities can result in double vision with different gaze directions. Therefore, during the assessment of eye movements, even subtle abnormalities can result in positional double vision. Because of this, the clinician should ask the patient about double vision with different positions of gaze. Assessing smooth-pursuit eye movements following TBI should also include the quality and speed of the movement. It is recommended to assess ocular movements in clockwise and counterclockwise motions. While doing so, it is important to carefully evaluate eye movements for sluggishness and nystagmus. During eye movement in a circular motion, the eye motion is passed from one muscle to another muscle at the 3-, 6-, 9-, and 12-o'clock positions. At these points during eye movement, the observer may notice a jump in eye movements because the motion is not smoothly passed from one muscle to another. It is also important to note any increase in symptoms with the testing described. Athletes who suffer visual problems following a concussion will most likely present with increased symptoms of headache, dizziness, and difficulty focusing with the testing described.

Pupillary Assessment

Pupil evaluation is equally important following TBI. Assessment regarding pupil reaction to both direct and indirect light should be performed. The Hippus response is not uncommon following mild TBI (mTBI) and may explain some of the sensitivity to light that patients experience following concussion. When testing for a Hippus response, the clinician will notice that the pupil will constrict then expand and constrict then expand when the light is directed at the eye. The Hippus response is by no means diagnostic of mTBI but is associated with central nervous system pathology.

Saccades

Evaluation of the eyes also includes assessing the quality of motion of saccadic eye movements. When assessing saccadic eye movement, it is important to assess both horizontally and vertically. The clinician should carefully observe eye motion and assess for sluggishness, deliberateness, and nystagmus. Many patients with visual dysfunction may experience symptoms of headache, dizziness, blurred or double vision, or head rush following saccadic eye movement testing. These patients also commonly express difficulty with their ability to rapidly move from one target to the next. They commonly refer to it as if their eyes are "sticking" or not able to move quickly. The saccadic eye movement should be more reflexive rather than deliberate.

Convergence Insufficiency

Convergence insufficiency (CI) is also a very common finding following acquired mTBI. The assessment of near point of convergence is a helpful tool in the diagnosis of CI. In assessing near point of convergence, the examiner has the patient focus on an object (the tip of the pin or focus stick). As the object is brought closer to the patient, the clinician evaluates how the eyes converge and the patient states when the object becomes double. A normal near point of convergence is 5 to 10 cm. Individuals with CI will report double vision at greater distances. The presence of abnormal near point of convergence on exam that persists over a significant period of time warrants a referral to a neuro-optometrist with experience in mTBI.

Vestibulo-Ocular Reflex

The assessment of the eyes also includes assessment of the vestibulo-ocular reflex (VOR). The VOR can be assessed in both the horizontal and vertical planes. The VOR can be assessed in a few ways. The clinician can sit in front of the patient and hold the patient's head and asks the patient to focus directly ahead on a stationary target (such as the clinician's nose). The clinician then moves the patient's head from side to side, slowly increasing the speed of head movement while watching to see if the patient can remain focused on the target. Some clinicians do this testing allowing the patient to actively move his or her head side to side while focusing directly ahead on a stationary target. The vertical VOR assessment is performed by repeating the same instructions but shaking the head up and down while the eyes remain fixed on the target. Following mTBI, patients with visual and/or vestibular dysfunction frequently experience symptoms of increased headache, dizziness, nausea, and difficulty focusing after these assessments. If the patient can tolerate increased head movement, the VOR can be more precisely assessed using the head thrust test (HTT). In this test, the clinician moves the patient's head side to side, slowly increasing the speed of head movement. If tolerated, the clinician then rapidly moves the patient's head once rapidly 20 to 30 degrees to either the right or the left. A patient with a normal VOR will maintain fixation on the target.[2] A patient with an impaired VOR will not be able to maintain fixation on the stationary target and will lose focus and then correct back to the target in a delayed fashion. This is called a corrective saccade. A patient with an abnormal VOR may become symptomatic with this testing, reporting difficulty focusing, dizziness, nausea, and increased headache. It is important to take into consideration any neck discomfort before performing the HTT.

Visual system and ocular movement disorders following concussion have been studied with increased frequency over the past few years and are an important part of the assessment protocol. The ocular movements mentioned previously are commonly affected with concussion and play a significant role in the recovery process. Any abnormalities in these tests can be treated through vestibular and functional vision therapy, and if symptoms persist or if visual problems do not improve, an evaluation from a neuro-optometrist specializing in mTBI is recommended. The combination of neuro-optometric rehabilitative therapy and vestibular and balance therapy is the most effective treatment for resolving these visual/vestibular symptoms related to concussion.[1]

References

1. Cohen A. Vision rehabilitation for visual-vestibular dysfunction: the role of the neuro-optometrist. *NeuroRehabilitation.* 2013;32:483-492.
2. Chandrasekhar S. The assessment of balance and dizziness in the TBI patient. *NeuroRehabilitation.* 2013;32:445-454.

HOW COMMON ARE VESTIBULAR DEFICITS FOLLOWING SPORT-RELATED CONCUSSION, AND WHAT TOOLS ARE BEST USED TO ASSESS VESTIBULAR DYSFUNCTION?

Shelly Massingale, PT, MPT

Vestibular and balance dysfunction after concussion are common, and the symptom of dizziness is one of the greatest predictors of a prolonged recovery. One study identified that athletes who have suffered a concussion on the field and immediately experienced dizziness were at greater risk of a prolonged recovery.[1] In order to understand, manage, and treat vestibular disorders related to concussion, it is important to utilize various tools to assess the vestibular system. It is also useful to divide treatment and management of vestibular deficits related to concussion into categories based on the onset of symptoms and length of time to resolution. Three major categories are commonly used for symptom duration: time after initial impact, recovery period, and prolonged recovery.[2]

Immediately following a sideline diagnosis of a concussion, the best treatment for the athlete is rest. The goal of treatment in the initial stage after impact is to allow healing to occur via withdrawal from physical and cognitive activities for a period of 24 hours.[3] After this initial rest period, the patient may have lasting symptoms of dizziness and/or visual problems. These symptoms are most often described as

Valovich McLeod TC, ed. *Quick Questions in Sport-Related Concussion: Expert Advice in Sports Medicine* (pp 85-90).
© 2015 Taylor & Francis Group.

a foggy feeling in the head, difficulty focusing, light sensitivity, and difficulty with reading tasks. If the patient suffers from vestibular symptoms (eg, dizziness, visual problems) after initial impact and after a period of rest, a more in-depth evaluation of the patient's symptoms can be valuable and could warrant vestibular rehabilitation to help with the recovery process. The time frame for this evaluation varies and is not clear in the research. It is very much dependent upon symptoms, history, and tolerance to certain stimuli. It is important to note that every concussion is different, so the management and treatment will vary depending on the symptoms and the patient's past medical history. Because vestibular evaluation and assessment can provoke the patient's symptoms, it is imperative to be aware of the patient's symptom levels, perhaps by administering a symptom scale, prior to administering any of the vestibular tests. Depending on the nature of the injury and intensity of symptoms, testing can be tolerated well, or it can be too provoking and contraindicated.

In order to assess the vestibular system in relationship to concussion, it is important to focus on all 3 balance systems: the somatosensory system, the vestibular system, and the visual system. Each system should be tested to determine pathology and functional impairment. Balance and vestibular dysfunction after a concussion can be caused by central vestibular deficits or peripheral vestibular deficits.[2] Testing done for both central and peripheral pathology can be performed in the clinical setting, and if needed, the athlete can be referred for more extensive testing of the central and peripheral vestibular systems by an audiologist or a physician who specializes in neuro-otology (disorders of the vestibular system). The following tools are used when assessing vestibular dysfunction in the clinic.

Benign Paroxysmal Position Vertigo

Benign paroxysmal position vertigo (BPPV) is usually the first related vestibular pathology to rule out.[2] BPPV is a peripheral vestibular disorder and is caused by free-floating calcium carbonate crystals in the semicircular canals, which cause a sensation of vertigo that occurs with positional changes.[4] BPPV is tested using the Dix-Hallpike test and is most commonly treated using the Canalith repositioning procedure. It is recommended that BPPV be treated by a trained clinician. Once BPPV is treated and/or ruled out, the following assessments should be performed.

Oculomotor Assessment

These tests are described in detail in Question 16. When assessing the oculomotor system, it is important for the clinician to not only focus on the quality of the eye movements but to also take note of the symptoms that the athlete reports while performing these tests.

Vestibulo-Ocular Reflex and Dynamic Visual Acuity

The primary function of the vestibular system is to maintain eye fixation on a target in the presence of head and body movement.[5] The vestibulo-ocular reflex (VOR) can be tested using the head thrust test (described in Question 16). Assessment of visual acuity during head movement can be done using a computerized system or in the clinic. Assessment of static and dynamic visual acuity in the clinic is done with a standard vision chart. The athlete is asked to sit in front of the vision chart and read the lowest line possible to determine static visual acuity (SVA) with both eyes. When testing dynamic visual acuity (DVA), the clinician stands behind the patient and shakes the patient's head from side to side 15 to 20 degrees each way at approximately 2 Hz, and the athlete is asked to read the lowest line on the vision chart. If the athlete can read the same line or up to 2 lines above it, it is considered a normal DVA test. Anything greater than 2 lines above SVA can be considered abnormal. An abnormal DVA test indicates difficulty with dynamic gaze stability. An athlete with an abnormal DVA could benefit from gaze stability exercises that focus on adaptation of the VOR.

Vestibulo-Ocular Reflex Supression

This test assesses the ability to suppress the VOR. It can be performed by having the athlete hold both arms straight out with thumbs up. The athlete focuses on the thumbs and rotates head and body enbloc while maintaining visual fixation on the thumbs. A normal VOR suppression test will show that the athlete is able to keep his or her eyes focused on the thumbs due to suppression of the VOR. If nystagmus is observed during rotation, it demonstrates impairment in VOR suppression. When testing VOR suppression in concussed athletes, it is very common for the athlete to have increased symptoms of dizziness, nausea, difficulty focusing, and difficulty maintaining balance when standing.

Static Balance Testing

Static balance testing is commonly performed using the Romberg and sharpened Romberg tests (standing with feet together and standing one foot in front of the other or heel to toe). Both testing positions are performed with eyes open and eyes closed on a noncompliant (firm) surface and on a compliant surface (foam). When performing these tests, the clinician evaluates the athlete's ability to maintain balance and measures the amount of sway in each testing situation. If force plate technology is available, the amount of sway can be measured objectively.

Neurovestibular Static Balance Testing

Neurovestibular (NVT) balance testing can be done to test the athlete's balance when directly stimulating the vestibular system by asking the athlete to shake his or her head side to side. This static balance test is done by asking the athlete to stand in Romberg position with eyes open and with eyes closed and perform head turns and head tilts to stimulate the vestibular system. This is done on both firm and foam surfaces. If the Romberg position is too difficult, the athlete is asked to stand with feet apart. Loss of balance and sway are recorded, as well as symptom provocation. These tests can also be done in the sharpened Romberg position on firm and foam surfaces for increased challenge.

Dynamic Balance Testing—Functional Gait Assessment

The functional gait assessment (FGA) is a functional balance test that is commonly used to test balance under dynamic situations (eg, walking with head turns/tilts, walking with eyes closed). With the FGA, the athlete is asked to do multiple tasks while walking, and each task is graded based on time of completion, loss of balance, and drifting/veering from a straight path.

Computerized Dynamic Posturography

Computerized dynamic posturography (CDP) evaluation is a helpful tool in assessing integration of visual, vestibular, and somatosensory information. Dynamic posturography is not a direct assessment of peripheral or central vestibular function but is a tool used to assess balance.[4] The most common balance function test in dynamic posturography is the Sensory Organization Test (SOT). The SOT assesses functional balance while challenging the visual, vestibular, and somatosensory systems. The SOT is performed with eyes open and eyes closed with the head still. If an athlete scores above normal on the SOT, the Head Shake SOT can be performed. With the Head Shake SOT, the clinician can evaluate balance function while stimulating the vestibular system through head movement. This is done without vision (eyes closed) and is on both a firm and a moving surface.

Videoelectronystagmography

If there is any reason that the clinician or physician feels that the athlete needs more extensive testing, it is common to refer to audiology services for videoelectronystagmography (VNG) testing. This testing can help identify peripheral versus central pathology. The VNG evaluation is a very helpful tool in the evaluation of a dizzy patient. The VNG assesses both peripheral and central inputs and includes smooth pursuits, saccade, and optokinetic testing with eye movement recordings and video-oculography.[6] The VNG also tests the function of the semicircular canals using water or air caloric testing.

Baseline Symptom Scores

Prior to performing a vestibular assessment, the most important role of the clinician is to determine baseline symptom scores that are directly related to vestibular dysfunction. These baseline scores are specifically related to how the patient is feeling at rest prior to beginning the activity or exercise that will be administered during that treatment session. Table 17-1 lists the most common vestibular symptoms following concussion: dizziness, nausea, visual problems/difficulty focusing, balance problems, headache, sensitivity to light/noise, and vertigo. Prior to performing the vestibular assessment, it is important to have the patient rate his or her symptoms on a scale of 0 to 10 in each of the categories listed. As the vestibular evaluation is performed, the clinician should continue to monitor the patient's symptoms compared with symptom report prior to that activity. The most difficult obstacle a clinician can come across when performing a vestibular evaluation is determining whether or not the testing or activity is too stimulating. For each vestibular test or activity that is performed, symptoms should be measured to determine the impact of the task on vestibular symptoms. When the activity is discontinued, it is recommended to have the patient sit and rest without any stimulation. If the patient's symptoms return to the level prior to the activity within 5 minutes of rest, the clinician can feel comfortable that the test or activity is appropriate. If the patient's symptoms do not return to the level prior to activity and remain elevated after 5 minutes, it is recommended to discontinue that activity or modify it to be less stimulating. When performing a vestibular evaluation, it is important to note what test procedures were too stimulating and to continue to monitor these activities during the management of the concussion.

Conclusion

Evaluating an athlete who has vestibular deficits is challenging due to the various symptoms and degrees of injury that can occur with this particular diagnosis. Even

Table 17-1

Common Vestibular Symptoms Related to Concussion

Symptom	Description
Dizziness	Sensation of feeling "off" or "foggy"; feeling "funny" in the head but not spinning
Nausea	Common symptom that occurs with dizziness, feeling of discomfort in the stomach
Visual problems/ difficulty focusing/ sensitivity to light	Difficulty with focusing with head movement, difficulty with vision in bright environments and visual sensitivity when moving in car, etc
Balance problems	Sensation of feeling off balance with activity, with walking, and with head movement
Headache	Feeling of pressure or dull ache in the head
Vertigo	True sensation of spinning, most commonly with positional changes

more challenging is the treatment and management of the athlete's symptoms once the testing is completed. It is most important to note that each concussion is different and that testing and treatment should focus on both objective testing results and on subjective report of symptoms. Vestibular testing and treatment is very effective in the recovery process for athletes with the diagnosis of concussion. With the appropriate tools and expert clinicians, this testing can help guide clinicians to make the best decisions on helping the athlete recover from vestibular deficits following concussion.

References

1. Lau BC, Collins MW, Lovell MR. Sensitivity and specificity of subacute computerized neurocognitive testing and symptom evaluation in predicting outcomes after sports-related concussion. *Am J Sports Med*. 2011;39(6):1209-1216.
2. Aligene K, Lin E. Vestibular and balance treatment of the concussed athlete. *NeuroRehabilitation*. 2013;32(3):543-553.
3. McCrory P, Meeuwisse W, Aubry M, et al. Consensus statement on concussion in sport: the 4th International Conference on Concussion in Sport held in Zurich, November 2012. *Clin J Sport Med*. 2013;23(2):89-117.
4. Herdman S. *Vestibular Rehabilitation*. 2nd ed. Philadelphia, PA: FA Davis Company; 2000.
5. Guskiewicz KM. Postural stability assessment following concussion: one piece of the puzzle. *Clin J Sport Med*. 2001;11:182-189.
6. Chandrasekhar SS. The assessment of balance and dizziness in the TBI patient. *NeuroRehabilitation*. 2013;32(3):445-454.

How Frequently and When Should Postconcussion Assessments Be Administered?

R.J. Elbin, PhD; Michael W. Collins, PhD; and
Anthony P. Kontos, PhD

Athletes with a concussion present with a wide range of signs, symptoms, and impairments that are heterogeneous. Due to this variability, it is recommended that the clinical assessment of concussion involve a comprehensive, multidimensional approach. Such an approach includes brief sideline assessments, symptom inventories, computerized neurocognitive test (CNT) batteries, and postural stability/balance assessments. Although this approach covers the many effects of concussion, it can also complicate the process of determining which assessments to use. In addition, there are the issues of when and how often to administer assessments following concussion. Some assessments are designed for use immediately following injury (ie, acute), whereas other assessments are designed to be used in the days and weeks following injury (ie, subacute). In this chapter, we will briefly introduce and review postconcussion administration practices for sideline concussion assessments, symptom inventories, and CNT batteries.

Valovich McLeod TC, ed. *Quick Questions in Sport-Related Concussion: Expert Advice in Sports Medicine* (pp 91-95).
© 2015 Taylor & Francis Group.

Sideline Assessment

The Sport Concussion Assessment Tool, 3rd Edition (SCAT3), is intended for the acute assessment of concussion. The SCAT3 includes cognitive components from the Standardized Assessment for Concussion (SAC) and measures of postural stability from the Balance Error Scoring System (BESS). The SAC is a brief cognitive assessment and neurological screening tool that assesses, in abbreviated fashion, symptoms and basic cognitive function, and the BESS is a noninstrumented assessment of postural stability. The SAC and BESS provide important data within the first day or two but are limited in their use beyond the acute postinjury period. Therefore, the SCAT3 is a valuable part of the comprehensive approach to the concussion assessment, especially on the sideline and perhaps in the first few days following injury; however, the SCAT3 is not intended for use in the subacute or office-based evaluation of concussion.

Symptom Inventories

Numerous concussion symptom inventories are available for the sports medicine professional (see Question 15). The Post-Concussion Symptom Scale (PCSS), Graded Symptom Checklist (GSC), and the Rivermead Post-Concussion Symptom Questionnaire all quantify the presence and severity of concussion symptoms. These tools are easy to administer and should be used throughout recovery from concussion (ie, acute, subacute, chronic). However, postconcussion symptom data are subjective because many athletes minimize their symptoms with the hopes of expediting their return to participation. These behaviors increase the complexity of the postconcussion assessment and support the use of more objective assessment methods such as neurocognitive testing.

Computerized Neurocognitive Testing

CNT is an integral part of a comprehensive assessment of concussion that measures several cognitive domains (eg, memory, learning, attention, reaction time). Typically, CNTs are administered at least 1 day following injury and can be used in conjunction with clinical exam/interview, symptom inventories, and vestibular and ocular motor assessments to manage recovery from concussion and inform clinical decision making. Ideally, CNTs are administered at preinjury (ie, baseline) and postinjury intervals, which allows for comparison of an athlete's postconcussion performance to his or her preinjury performance. Although normative data are available for comparison in the absence of a baseline, obtaining a baseline measure

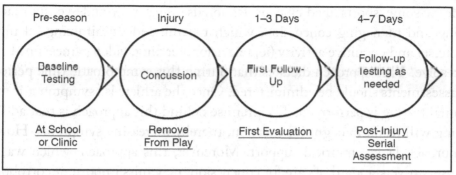

Figure 18-1. Recommended postconcussion assessment approach for the sports medicine professional. Documenting concussion signs/signs/symptoms, both on-field (ie, on-field dizziness) and within 1 week of injury (ie, posttraumatic migraine symptoms), are predictive of protracted recovery. Using computerized neuro-cognitive testing within the first week of concussion can also identify athletes at risk of prolonged recovery and inform management interventions (eg, academic accommodations). Serial assessments should be readministered every 7 days thereafter until the athlete is asymptomatic and back to baseline.

of neurocognitive performance is recommended. We liken the use of baseline CNT to measures of blood pressure, heart rate, and body mass index that are obtained by primary care physicians during routine checkups. The goal of these measures is to provide clinicians with a comparison to determine if an athlete is not within "normal limits" relative to his or her own individual healthy levels.

There are several CNT batteries available that include the Immediate Post-Concussion Assessment and Cognitive Testing (ImPACT), CNS Vital Signs, Headminder, and CogState Sport. These batteries comprise several versions and stimuli sets that help minimize practice effects and allow these tools to be read-ministered several times throughout the recovery from concussion. While the postconcussion testing schedule varies on a case-by-case basis, general postconcussion testing recommendations for CNT include initial testing at 24 to 72 hours postconcussion and weekly thereafter until the athlete performs at or near baseline levels (Figure 18-1).

When and How Often Should Athletes Be Tested Following a Concussion?

There is debate among clinicians and researchers about the frequency and timing of the administration of CNT following concussion, especially when the athlete is symptomatic. Self-reported symptoms remain the centerpiece of the concussion evaluation, and when the concussed athlete is still reporting increased symptoms, he or she is still considered injured and should not be permitted to return to play.

Therefore, some sports medicine professionals use a wait-and-see approach for assessing and managing concussion, which recommends minimizing all physical (ie, exercise) and cognitive activity (ie, television, reading, video games) until symptoms resolve. This approach dictates that during this symptomatic time period, no other assessments should be administered. Once the athlete is asymptomatic at rest, additional testing is performed. The premise behind this approach is that additional testing will result in cognitive exertion, thereby increasing symptoms. However, this approach lacks empirical support. Moreover, this approach, which was once the conservative standard of care for concussion, may miss important corroborative and prognostic information about the injury that may be used to expedite recovery.

In contrast to the wait-and-see approach is the serial postconcussion assessment of both symptoms and neurocognitive performance at regular postinjury time intervals. This assessment approach typically includes assessing symptoms at the time of injury using an on-field measure, which is then followed by a CNT and an assessment of symptoms 24 to 72 hours after injury. Additional follow-up testing for both symptoms and neurocognitive performance is then completed at approximately 5- to 7-day intervals until the athlete returns to, or near, baseline levels. This evidence-based approach[1] improves clinical accuracy for management decisions. Data obtained with this protocol inform management (eg, academic accommodations) and rehabilitation strategies. For example, school personnel might provide academic accommodations for an athlete with lingering memory deficits on CNT and symptoms of fogginess and difficulty concentrating. In addition, frequent assessment of symptoms and neurocognitive performance provides important feedback for the concussed athlete. These tools provide tangible evidence of improvement, which increase the concussed athlete's sense of control in an often ambiguous and unclear recovery period. Postconcussion symptom reports and neurocognitive performance should complement each other because any disparity between these sources of information should be addressed.

Assessing postconcussion symptoms and neurocognitive performance within the first week following concussion is supported strongly in the literature and has several clinical advantages. Assessing both symptoms and neurocognitive performance within the first 2 to 3 days of concussion improves the diagnostic yield (ie, correctly diagnosing concussion) to 93%, which is higher than using only symptoms (64% of concussions accurately detected) and CNTs alone (83% of concussions accurately identified).[2] Clinicians can also predict approximately 73% of the time that an athlete will take longer than 1 month to recover based on CNT and symptom data obtained within the acute time period following concussion.[3] Assessing symptoms within 7 days of injury also has prognostic value because certain symptom subgroups such as posttraumatic migraine (headache, nausea, and sensitivity to light and/or noise) are a significant predictor of longer recovery times and more pronounced impairment.[4] Symptom assessments obtained within 7 days of concussion reveal that most athletes report a predominantly global cognitive-fatigue-migraine cluster of symptoms,[5] and after a few weeks these symptoms typically shift into more well-defined affective, cognitive, somatic, and sleep symptom clusters. Understanding the relationship between symptom reports and CNT data obtained in the acute and subacute phases following injury will ultimately improve the clinical management of sport-related concussion.

References

1. Collins M, Lovell MR, Iverson GL, Ide T, Maroon J. Examining concussion rates and return to play in high school football players wearing newer helmet technology: a three-year prospective cohort study. *Neurosurgery.* 2006;58(2):275-286.
2. Van Kampen DA, Lovell MR, Pardini JE, Collins MW, Fu FH. The "value added" of neurocognitive testing after sports-related concussion. *Am J Sports Med.* 2006;34(10):1630-1635.
3. Lau BC, Collins MW, Lovell MR. Sensitivity and specificity of subacute computerized neurocognitive testing and symptom evaluation in predicting outcomes after sports-related concussion. *Am J Sports Med.* 2011;39(6):1209-1216.
4. Kontos AP, Elbin RJ, Lau B, et al. Posttraumatic migraine as a predictor of recovery and cognitive impairment after sport-related concussion. *Am J Sports Med.* 2013;41(7):1497-1504.
5. Kontos AP, Elbin RJ, Schatz P, et al. A revised factor structure for the post-concussion symptom scale: baseline and postconcussion factors. *Am J Sports Med.* 2012;40(10):2375-2384.

DOES RECOVERY ON CLINICAL TESTS REPRESENT TRUE RECOVERY OF THE BRAIN?

Steven P. Broglio, PhD, ATC and Douglas Martini, MS

The diagnosis of concussion and the return-to-play (RTP) decision should be completed on a case-by-case basis, with the clinical examination serving as the gold standard for both injury phases. Because management of the injury in both phases is a subjective process, considerable research efforts have been devoted to developing and validating tools that provide objective information to the clinician. A number of sports medicine groups support the use of objective tools, with measures of athlete-reported symptoms, postural control, and neurocognitive function being the most common.[1]

When a baseline evaluation of the athlete is available, tests for each of these domains (ie, symptoms, balance, and neurocognitive function) are approximately 60% sensitive to acute deficits following injury but when combined offer sensitivity greater than 90%. In most concussion cases, the athlete's reports of symptoms are monitored on a daily basis, and balance and neurocognitive assessments are readministered once the athlete no longer reports concussion-related symptoms. If the athlete demonstrates a return to preinjury/baseline levels of postural control and

Valovich McLeod TC, ed. *Quick Questions in Sport-Related Concussion: Expert Advice in Sports Medicine* (pp 97-99).
© 2015 Taylor & Francis Group.

neurocognitive function, an RTP progression is begun following a normal clinical examination. However, what remains largely unknown is if the athlete's performance on these tests represents complete metabolic recovery from the injury or a return to a functional level of performance, despite ongoing cellular-level recovery that is not detectable by current clinical tests.

The return-to-baseline levels of function on measures of self-reported symptoms, postural control, and neurocognitive performance are well documented. For example, collegiate-level athletes with a concussion are reported to return to preinjury levels of balance between days 3 and 5 postinjury, while cognitive function and symptoms return by day 7.[2] Following this acute stage of injury, an RTP progression lasting up to 1 week is often implemented. In most cases, concussed athletes are withheld from full sport participation for 10 to 14 days following the injury. However, modern research tools are being implemented in this area to discern between function recovery and true metabolic recovery of concussed athletes. Although these measures are not typically seen in clinical settings, the results are compelling.

Magnetic resonance imaging (MRI) has been implemented in the sporting environment for a number of years and has proven invaluable for orthopedic injuries. An adjunct methodology—functional MRI (fMRI)—is now being used as a tool that measures areas of brain activation during a cognitive task or stimulus. In one investigation of collegiate-level football athletes,[3] fMRI evaluations were administered prior to the competitive season, along with standard neurocognitive assessments (ie, Digit Span and Addition and Subtraction tests). During the season, 4 athletes sustained diagnosed concussions and were evaluated within 1 week of the injury, along with 4 control/noninjured athletes. The results showed, as expected, that the concussed and control athletes performed equally on the neurocognitive assessments. However, the concussed athletes continued to show higher levels of cerebral activation on the postinjury fMRI assessment relative to the control athletes and their own baseline. The authors concluded that the concussed athletes recruited additional cortical resources in order to perform at the same functional level as the control athletes, despite ongoing metabolic changes.[3] Another investigation of concussed athletes evaluated cerebral metabolism following injury by implementing magnetic resonance spectroscopy (MRS). Alterations to cerebral metabolism are a well-known effect of concussion as the brain escalates energy demand to restore the ionic imbalance brought about by the impact.[4] When concussed athletes were evaluated using MRS, the scans indicated that cerebral metabolism did not return to noninjured levels until between 22 and 30 days postinjury, despite symptom resolution between days 3 and 15.[5]

Ultimately, it appears that the combined use of concussion assessments commonly implemented in clinical settings are sensitive to cerebral declines. However, these same tests may not provide the requisite sensitivity to detect ongoing subtle changes beyond the 7- to 10-day window that is the normal recovery time course. As such, to believe that an individual has achieved "complete" recovery based on a return to baseline scores on clinical tests may be inaccurate. These new findings parallel what is known about orthopedic injuries. For example, an athlete with a bone fracture may be functional within 6 to 8 weeks, but complete healing takes place over the next year. What is less clear is how these findings translate to clinical practice. As is the case with the majority of sports-related injuries, the athlete is released to return to the field when he or she becomes functional. There are known risks for doing this, but how this relates to short- and long-term cognitive health is less clear.

References

1. Broglio SP, Cantu RC, Gioia GA, et al. NATA position statement on the management of sport concussion. *J Athl Train*. 2014;49(2):245-265.
2. McCrea M, Guskiewicz KM, Marshall SW, et al. Acute effects and recovery time following concussion in collegiate football players: the NCAA Concussion Study. *JAMA*. 2003;290:2556-2563.
3. Jantzen KJ, Anderson B, Steinberg FL, Kelso JA. A prospective functional MR imaging study of mild traumatic brain injury in college football players. *Am J Neuroradiol*. 2004;25:738-745.
4. Giza CC, Hovda DA. The neurometabolic cascade of concussion. *J Athl Train*. 2001;36:228-235.
5. Vagnozzi R, Signoretti S, Cristofori L, et al. Assessment of metabolic brain damage and recovery following mild traumatic brain injury: a multicentre, proton magnetic resonance spectroscopic study in concussed patients. *Brain*. 2010;133:3232-3242.

IS IMAGING USEFUL TO DETERMINE THE SEVERITY OF, OR THE TIME TO RECOVERY FROM, A CONCUSSION?

Max Zeiger, BS; Meeryo C. Choe, MD; and
Christopher C. Giza, MD

A concussion as defined by the International Conference on Concussion in Sports is "a complex pathophysiological process affecting the brain, induced by biomechanical forces. A concussion may be caused by a direct blow to the head, face, neck, or elsewhere on the body and typically results in the rapid onset of short-lived impairment of neurological function."[1] These short-lived impairments are functional disturbances in the brain rather than structural injuries. Therefore, abnormalities cannot generally be detected using standard structural neuroimaging studies.[2]

Imaging for Concussion Diagnosis

When evaluating an athlete who has sustained a concussion, it is important to determine when imaging is necessary because it can be used to detect more serious injuries such as intracranial hemorrhage or skull fracture. Frequently, computed tomography (CT) scans are obtained in children and adults who have sustained

Valovich McLeod TC, ed. *Quick Questions in Sport-Related Concussion: Expert Advice in Sports Medicine* (pp 101-104).
© 2015 Taylor & Francis Group.

a mild traumatic brain injury (mTBI). However, only a very small percentage of patients with concussions show intracranial injury on CT. Reducing the unnecessary use of CT scans is important to minimize the risk of exposure to ionizing radiation, particularly in children.[3]

In an analysis of 42,412 children presenting with head trauma in 25 US emergency departments (EDs), a clinical prediction rule was derived and validated to help stratify patients based on the risk of clinically important TBI (ciTBI).[4] CiTBI was defined as any TBI visible on CT that resulted in death, neurosurgery, intubation (more than 24 hours), or hospitalization (more than 2 nights). For children aged older than 2 years, if they presented to the ED with a Glasgow Coma Scale (GCS) score lower than 14, altered mental status, or palpable skull fracture, the risk of ciTBI was 4.4% and CT was recommended. If the patient did not meet these criteria, a second screening was based on history of loss of consciousness, vomiting, severe headache, or severe mechanism of injury (including severe motor vehicle accident, cyclist or pedestrian struck by motor vehicle, a fall of less than 1.5 m, or having the head struck by high-impact object). For patients with one of these clinical factors, the risk of ciTBI was 0.9%, and either observation or CT scanning could be utilized. Patients without any of these clinical characteristics at the time of ED presentation had a less than 0.05% risk of ciTBI and CT scanning was *not* recommended. In general, CT scanning was not recommended to rule out concussion, but only when more serious intracranial injury was suspected.

Evidence-based CT imaging guidelines for adult TBI have also been developed.[5] For patients with mTBI/concussion who present to the ED, a noncontrast head CT scan is indicated for those with loss of consciousness (LOC) or posttraumatic amnesia (PTA) if one or more of the following is present: headache, vomiting, age older than 60 years, drug/alcohol intoxication, short-term memory deficits, physical evidence of trauma above clavicle, posttraumatic seizure, GCS score lower than 15, focal neurological deficit, or coagulopathy (level A recommendation). For patients with no LOC or PTA, CT scanning may be considered if there is a focal neurological deficit, vomiting, severe headache, age older than 65 years, basilar skull fracture, GCS score lower than 15, coagulopathy, or severe mechanism of injury (level B).

Imaging to Determine Recovery

Concussions are complex injuries that result in a series of neurometabolic events within the brain, with distinct phases of injury and recovery. These phases have been detected using advanced neuroimaging techniques, including positron emission tomography (PET), magnetic resonance spectroscopy (MRS), and diffusion tensor imaging (DTI), and may provide insight into the recovery time from a concussion.[2]

[18]F-fluorodeoxyglucose (FDG)-PET scans, which measure cerebral glucose metabolism, have been used in studies to detect glucose metabolic depression following TBI.[4] In moderate and severe TBI, metabolic recovery takes weeks to months to return to baseline levels.[6] FDG-PET studies after mTBI/concussion have also shown profound glucose metabolic depression. However, longitudinal studies following concussion have yet to be done, and so the time period of dysfunction for this is not known.

Magnetic resonance imaging (MRI) has also been studied increasingly in the evaluation of mTBI/concussion. In an ED study that utilized both CT and MRI scanning of 135 mTBI patients (age older than 15 years), the presence of brain contusions or 4 or more foci of hemorrhagic axonal injury on structural MRI were each independently associated with poorer 3-month outcomes (4.5-fold and 3.2-fold, respectively).[7]

MRS, an advanced MRI technique that measures key brain metabolites, has shown diminished signal for *N*-acetylaspartate (NAA) in concussed athletes who took 30 days to return to baseline. Interestingly, athletes who sustained a second concussion prior to full recovery showed lower NAA levels acutely and took longer (45 days) to recover to baseline.[8] Such NAA abnormalities may indicate a period of metabolic vulnerability within the brain, but the correlation between abnormal NAA levels and clinical signs and symptoms is not clear. In this study, athletes were reportedly asymptomatic by postinjury day 3, but no systematic concussion assessment was documented at each time point.

Another advanced imaging tool that may provide insight into recovery time following concussion is DTI, which measures the directionality of water diffusion and has been used to evaluate axonal/white matter integrity. Fractional anisotropy (FA) is a measure of the orientation of water diffusion—the higher the FA, the more directional the water diffusion and, by inference, the more intact the white matter fibers. Lower FA has been correlated with reduced axonal integrity. However, following TBI, DTI results have been challenging to interpret. In some studies, increases in FA correlate with early clinical postinjury concussion symptoms.[9] Other studies also show increases in FA early after TBI, but these increases persist long after symptoms have resolved.[10] Still other reports show decreased FA following TBI and even after head contact exposure.[11,12]

Conclusion

CT scanning is currently not recommended to diagnose concussion but is useful to distinguish and diagnose more severe TBI such as hemorrhage, contusion, or skull fracture. While advanced neuroimaging such as PET or MRI has shown promise in distinguishing concussed from control athletes in a research setting, the use of advanced MRI for clinical management of individual patients is premature. More study is needed to determine how to best utilize newer imaging modalities to diagnose or to determine the time to recovery after TBI.

References

1. McCrory P, Meeuwisse WH, Aubry M, et al. Consensus statement on concussion in sport: the 4th International Conference on Concussion in Sport held in Zurich, November 2012. *Br J Sports Med*. 2013;47(5):250-258.
2. Di Fiori JP, Giza CC. New techniques in concussion imaging. *Curr Sports Med Rep*. 2010;9(1):35-39.
3. Brenner DJ, Hall EJ. Computed tomography: an increasing source of radiation exposure. *N Engl J Med*. 2007;357(22):2277-2284.
4. Kuppermann N, Holmes JF, Dayan PS, et al. Identification of children at very low risk of clinically-important brain injuries after head trauma: a prospective cohort study. *Lancet*. 2009;374(9696):1160-1170.
5. Jagoda AS, Bazarian JJ, Bruns JJ Jr, et al. Clinical policy: neuroimaging and decision making in adult mild traumatic brain injury in the acute setting. *Ann Emerg Med*. 2008;52(6):714-748.
6. Bergsneider M, Hovda DA, McArthur DL, et al. Metabolic recovery following human traumatic brain injury based on FDG-PET: time course and relationship to neurological disability. *J Head Trauma Rehabil*. 2001;16(2):135-148.
7. Yuh EL, Mukherjee P, Lingsma HF, et al. Magnetic resonance imaging improves 3-month outcome prediction in mild traumatic brain injury. *Ann Neurol*. 2013;73(2):224-235.
8. Vagnozzi R, Signoretti S, Tavazzi B, et al. Temporal window of metabolic brain vulnerability to concussion: a pilot 1H-magnetic resonance spectroscopic study in concussed athletes—part III. *Neurosurgery*. 2008;62(6):1286-1295.
9. Wilde EA, McCauley SR, Hunter JV, et al. Diffusion tensor imaging of acute mild traumatic brain injury in adolescents. *Neurology*. 2008;70(12):948-955.
10. Mayer AR, Ling JM, Yang Z, Pena A, Yeo RA, Klimaj S. Diffusion abnormalities in pediatric mild traumatic brain injury. *J Neurosci*. 2012;32(50):17961-17969.
11. Lipton ML, Kim N, Zimmerman ME, et al. Soccer heading is associated with white matter microstructural and cognitive abnormalities. *Radiology*. 2013;268(3):850-857.
12. Strain J, Didehbani N, Cullum CM, et al. Depressive symptoms and white matter dysfunction in retired NFL players with concussion history. *Neurology*. 2013;81(1):25-32.

SECTION IV

CONCUSSION MANAGEMENT CONSIDERATIONS

SHOULD CONCUSSIONS IN CHILDREN AND ADOLESCENTS BE MANAGED DIFFERENTLY FROM THOSE IN ADULTS?

Richelle M. Williams, MS, ATC and
Tamara C. Valovich McLeod, PhD, ATC, FNATA

Proper management is an integral part of the recovery process following a concussion. Concussions can occur at any age and in any setting. There are recommendations on the management of concussion that span all ages[1,2]; however, extra care should be taken in regard to recovery when managing children and adolescents. There are many factors that place younger individuals at risk for concussions and age-specific postinjury sequelae that require different management tactics than those for adults.

Several structural and functional differences exist between the brain of a child and that of an adult. These include a thinner skull and proportionally larger head compared to the body in children, alterations in the need for glucose, decreased myelination, and increased blood flow. While it has yet to be determined which structural or functional differences factor into the differences noted between children, adolescents, and adults, any of these or a combination of several may be responsible.

Valovich McLeod TC, ed. *Quick Questions in Sport-Related Concussion: Expert Advice in Sports Medicine* (pp 107-111).
© 2015 Taylor & Francis Group.

An important concern with an unreported concussion or improper management is the possibility of premature return to play and the potential for second-impact syndrome. This condition is described as rapid swelling and vascular engorgement of the brain following a second impact to the head or elsewhere in the body while the brain is still recovering from the first injury.[3] Often, a concussion may not be reported and an athlete continues to participate with symptoms. A second force to the head or to the body that results in the transfer of force to the head can lead to immediate brain swelling and catastrophic outcomes, with a 50% mortality rate and 100% morbidity rate.[3] While this is a rare condition, it seems to primarily occur in athletes younger than 18 years, and little can be done to prevent the catastrophic consequences once the second impact has happened. Fortunately, proper management of the first concussion is the key. This includes proper assessment of the young athlete and conservative management through the return-to-play progression.

Baseline or preseason testing in the child or adolescent is an area of debate. The American Academy of Neurology[4] indicates there is insufficient use for the baseline model in the preadolescent, and the Zurich recommendations[1] suggest there is not enough evidence to promote the use of widespread baseline testing. Further complicating the matter is the ongoing development of cognition and balance in this age group, which would likely require baseline testing to be done at least on an annual basis to ensure appropriate scores are available for comparison to any postinjury test. Therefore, it is not common for children to have baseline data available.

The initial assessment of a child or adolescent is necessary to determine the nature and severity of symptoms, as well as any cognitive or balance deficits. A multifaceted approach to concussion assessment is still advocated, although the tools need to be tailored for the developmental age of the patient being evaluated.[5] One good example is the recently developed Child Sport Concussion Assessment Tool, 3rd Edition (Child SCAT3),[1] which was developed to evaluate concussion in children aged 5 to 12 years. The tool includes both patient and parent symptom inventories, a brief cognitive assessment, balance evaluation, and coordination test. The wording of the instrument is aimed at the intended patient population with the use of phrases to describe symptoms, rather than simply presenting a list of symptoms. Should clinicians want to use additional assessments, such as computerized neurocognitive tests, it is important to identify that the tool is intended and appropriate for that patient. There are many paper-and-pencil neurocognitive tests that have been well validated in children and adolescents that can be administered and interpreted by a neuropsychologist. Table 21-1 provides appropriate age ranges for some commonly used sport-concussion assessment tools.

Recovery following a concussion is another component that should be altered based on age. Previous research has shown that adolescents take longer to recover

Table 21-1

Cognitive and Balance Assessment Tools for Children and Adolescents

Assessment Tool	Type of Assessment	Domain Assessed	Appropriate Age Range
ImPACT	Computerized neurocognitive	Symptoms, verbal and visual memory, reaction time, and processing speed	Website indicates norms available for ages 10 to 59 years; most often used in patients > 13 years
Axon Sports Computerized Cognitive Assessment Tool (CCAT)	Computerized neurocognitive	Processing speed, attention, learning and working memory	> 10 years
Concussion Vital Signs	Computerized neurocognitive	Memory, psychomotor speed, executive function, cognitive flexibility, continuous performance task, reaction time	Website indicates norms available for ages 8 to 90 years
SCAT3	Multifaceted paper assessment	Symptoms, mental status (orientation, immediate and delayed memory, concentration), balance, coordination	> 13 years
Child SCAT3	Multifaceted paper assessment	Symptoms (patient self-report and parent-proxy), mental status (orientation, immediate and delayed memory, concentration), balance, coordination	5 to 12 years
Balance Error Scoring System (BESS)	Clinical balance assessment	Balance	Studies have administered the BESS to children as young as 9 years
Sensory Organization Test	Computerized balance assessment	Balance	Normative data available for ages ≥3 years

from concussions than college athletes and therefore management should be more conservative.[6,7] Due to the developmental stages of an adolescent, it is important to modify cognitive rest, physical rest, and school integration to be age appropriate. Cognitive and physical rest demands are different between adults and adolescents. Because an adolescent brain is still developing, it is important to take caution to avoid returning a participant back to sports or reintegrating him or her into academics too soon.[8,9] It is important to approach cautiously when returning adolescents to the classroom. There are steps that can be taken to help facilitate cognitive recovery for adolescents in regards to school, and these are discussed in more detail in later chapters. Adolescents experiencing severe symptoms should not attend school immediately following a concussion; however, if arrangements cannot be made to leave the student at home, accommodations should be made for that student. Some accommodations include excused absence; longer time for testing, homework, and projects; breaks throughout the school day; and accommodations for noise and light sensitivity.[9] In addition, a return-to-learn progression should be followed to progressively increase academic demands as tolerated.

Return to activity should follow a progression of increasing demands beginning once symptoms have resolved at rest.[1] This progression should be individualized and may be longer than those used in adult patients. Prior to any discussion of returning to physical activity and sports, patients should be able to tolerate a full day in the classroom without any academic accommodations. Patients should be evaluated on a daily basis throughout the progression to ensure that symptoms do not return with increased physical demands. The progression should also require at least one contact practice prior to full clearance for participation in games or competition.

Conclusion

A concussion to an adolescent brain that is still developing can be dangerous and requires early recognition and effective management to reduce the risk of more serious conditions or a prolonged recovery. It is necessary to have age-appropriate assessment tools to assess total range of symptoms, neurocognitive functions, and balance, as well as management guidelines for adolescent athletes, which incorporate the oversight of parental involvement with management of returning to sports as well as school and home functioning.

References

1. McCrory P, Meeuwisse W, Aubry M, et al. Consensus statement on concussion in sport: the 4th International Conference on Concussion in Sport held in Zurich, November 2012. *Clin J Sport Med.* 2013;23(2):89-117.
2. Broglio SP, Cantu RC, Gioia GA, et al. National Athletic Trainers' Association position statement on the management of sport-related concussion update. *J Athl Train.* 2014;49(2):245-265.
3. Cantu RC. Second impact syndrome. *Clin Sport Med.* 1998;17(1):37-43.
4. Giza CC, Kutcher JS, Ashwal S, et al. Summary of evidence-based guideline update: evaluation and management of concussion in sports: report of the Guideline Development Subcommittee of the American Academy of Neurology. *Neurology.* 2013;80(24):2250-2257.
5. Guskiewicz KM, Valovich McLeod TC. Pediatric sports-related concussion. *PM R.* 2011;3(4):353-364.
6. Field M, Collins MW, Lovell MR, Maroon JC. Does age play a role in recovery from sports-related concussion? A comparison of high school and collegiate athletes. *J Pediatr.* 2003;142:546-553.
7. Sim A, Terryberry-Spohr L, Wilson KR. Prolonged recovery of memory functioning after mild traumatic brain injury in adolescent athletes. *J Neurosurg.* 2008;108(3):511-516.
8. Halstead ME, Walter KD. American Academy of Pediatrics. Clinical report: sport-related concussion in children and adolescents. *Pediatrics.* 2010;126(3):597-615.
9. Halstead ME, McAvoy K, Devore CD, Carl R, Lee M, Logan K. Returning to learning following a concussion. *Pediatrics.* 2013;132(5):948-957.

HOW MANY CONCUSSIONS ARE TOO MANY BEFORE AN ATHLETE SHOULD RETIRE?

Amaal J. Starling, MD; Meeryo C. Choe, MD; and Christopher C. Giza, MD

Concussion is a clinical syndrome characterized by acute, but generally transient, neurologic impairment due to biomechanical forces imparted to the brain. The most commonly reported symptom is headache, although cognitive impairment, amnesia, disequilibrium, sleep disturbances, and behavioral changes are frequently reported as well. By definition, these neurologic symptoms and signs should recover with time; however, there is growing concern for irreversible cumulative effects of repeat concussions. This raises the clinical question that we will address in this chapter—how many concussions are too many before an athlete should retire? Three clinical presentations that should prompt the treating clinician to recommend retirement from contact sports include the following: (1) diagnosis of a neurodegenerative condition, (2) permanent or persistent cognitive or neurobehavioral impairment, and (3) intractable pain and headache (Table 22-1). A relative indication to consider retirement would be progressively lower threshold for concussion with worse symptoms. We will address the evidence that supports these conclusions.

Valovich McLeod TC, ed. *Quick Questions in Sport-Related Concussion: Expert Advice in Sports Medicine* (pp 113-118).
© 2015 Taylor & Francis Group.

Table 22-1
Four Clinical Presentations That Should Prompt Recommendations for Retirement From Contact Sports
Strongly recommend retirement if there is:
Diagnosis of a neurodegenerative condition
Permanent or persistent cognitive or neurobehavioral impairment
Intractable pain and headache
Consider recommending retirement if there is:
Progressively lower threshold for concussion or progressively more severe symptoms

Neurodegeneration

The risk of developing a neurodegenerative condition such as Alzheimer's disease, Parkinson's disease, or amyotrophic lateral sclerosis is of paramount concern for athletes and their families. A recent community-based study with 50-year follow-up found no difference in the development of dementia or other neurodegenerative conditions between athletes that played football in high school and their band member classmates.[1] However, Lehman et al demonstrated that retired National Football League players have a neurodegenerative mortality that is 3 times higher than that of the general US population.[2] These data suggest that the level of play (amateur vs professional) may influence the risk of developing a neurodegenerative condition.

Chronic traumatic encephalopathy (CTE) is a pathologically described progressive tauopathy, with associated symptoms of cognitive and behavioral decline. CTE has been found in several professional and amateur athletes and has been associated with a history of repetitive brain trauma. However, currently published studies are limited to case reports and case series. These studies may demonstrate the occurrence of the disorder but are unable to determine the prevalence, incidence, or risk factors associated with CTE. Most importantly, causation remains unclear. Repeat concussions, repeat subconcussive hits, and/or genetic vulnerability could play a major role in the development of CTE but are as yet unproven.

- Presentation: A clinical diagnosis of a neurodegenerative condition, including Alzheimer's disease, Parkinson's disease, other dementia, or amyotrophic lateral sclerosis, should prompt a health care provider to recommend retirement from contact sports. Currently, it is not possible to definitively diagnose CTE antemortem, but if an athlete begins to show commonly associated clinical symptoms and signs of cognitive and behavioral decline, a discussion of retirement is reasonable.

Chronic or Persistent Neurocognitive Impairment

Chronic neurocognitive and neurobehavioral impairment has been associated with a history of repeated concussions or prolonged exposure to contact sports. Retired professional football players reporting a history of 3 or more concussions had a 5-fold increased prevalence of mild cognitive impairment compared with retired athletes reporting no history of concussions.[3] Cognitive impairment can be objectively quantified with comprehensive neuropsychometric testing. Recent data suggest a decrease in verbal memory scores after 3 or more concussions on comprehensive neuropsychometric testing.

In fact, multiple studies of professional athletes in football, soccer, rugby, horseracing, and boxing have shown objective cognitive impairment during life when measured using neuropsychological testing. All of these studies in professionals also showed evidence for a dose response; namely, athletes with a greater measure of exposure to brain impacts showed a larger degree of cognitive impairment.[4-6] Although a strong relationship between chronic cognitive impairments has been seen in multiple professional sports, similar studies in amateur athletes (high school, collegiate, adult amateurs) have been inconclusive.[7]

Several well-known professional athletes have suffered from depression and committed suicide. This has been widely covered by the press, and repeat concussive injuries have been implicated. Recent questionnaire data have demonstrated increased risk of depression (but not suicidality) with the higher number of self-reported concussions in a dose-dependent manner.[8,9]

- Presentation: Permanent or persistent cognitive impairment (memory, executive dysfunction) or neurobehavioral problems (such as depression, anxiety) should prompt consideration for a contact/collision sports athlete to retire. These risks appear greatest in professional boxing, football, rugby, soccer, and horseracing. Preexisting learning disabilities and psychiatric comorbidities complicate the evaluation of these athletes. In most cases, obtaining objective evidence of persistent neurocognitive impairment is warranted for making retirement from contact/collision sport decisions.

Chronic or Intractable Headache or Pain

Frequent, severe headaches have been correlated with repeat concussive injuries in both high school and collegiate athletes. Some athletes may have preexisting headache disorders that are exacerbated by concussions. In fact, athletes with a history of migraine are susceptible to more severe, chronic headaches after head injury.[10]

- Presentation: If repetitive concussions result in an escalating severity, chronicity, or intractability of headache or pain, retirement from contact/collision sports should be considered.

Reduced Threshold for and/or Increasing Severity of Concussion

Some athletes who have suffered from repeat concussions appear to develop a reduced threshold of inducing injury. In these situations, seemingly mild biomechanical forces to the head result in loss of consciousness or prolonged postconcussive symptoms. Strong prospective evidence indicates increased risk for concussion in those with prior concussions and that this risk is greatest within the first 7 to 10 days after a concussion. There is evidence that suggests repeated concussions can be more severe or have more persistent symptoms.[11,12]

- Presentation: If an athlete demonstrates a pattern of lower threshold to develop concussion symptoms and/or greater/more prolonged symptoms after repeated concussions, retirement from contact sports should be discussed.

So, how do we counsel our athletes? Due to the many variables involved, there will not be a cutoff number for the number of concussions that will automatically prompt a health care provider to recommend retirement to an athlete. A health care provider will need to synthesize the complicated clinical scenario, starting with a detailed history, taking into consideration age, sex, prior concussion/traumatic brain injury, preexisting conditions, sport, player position, style of play, and cumulative exposure to contact risk.

Due to underreporting and underdiagnosis of concussions and recent evidence for long-term sequelae of subconcussive hits, estimation of exposure should not be limited to number of concussions but also include a discussion and consideration of duration of participation, level of participation (starter vs reserve), number of practices/games, and even biomechanical sensor data if available.

When evaluating an athlete for the cumulative effects of concussion, beyond the clinical history, a careful neurologic exam is critical. Such an assessment should include careful examination for mental status impairments, cranial neuropathies, dysarthria, incoordination, bradykinesia, increased tone, ataxia, tremor, hyper-reflexia, and "soft" neurological signs. Additional tools may be needed, including comprehensive neuropsychometric testing and neuroimaging. Many of these can only be performed by a neurologist in consultation with other health care providers.

Evidence of dementia, neurodegeneration, permanent/persistent cognitive or neurobehavioral impairment, or intractable headache/pain strongly supports retirement from contact sports, particularly for high-exposure professional athletes. Although the number of concussions is important, there is no set number of concussions that mandates retirement, and other important factors should be considered before making the recommendation for retirement. Ultimately, each retirement decision will be highly individualized, taking into account any advantages of continued play (income, professional advancement, fitness) vs disadvantages and potential risks (chronic cognitive, behavioral, or pain-related symptoms).

Conclusion

Although the symptoms and signs following an individual concussion are generally fully reversible, persistent neurologic impairment is a concern after repeated concussions. There is no simple algorithm to determine how many concussions are too many, and one may even question whether counting concussions should give way to other estimates of contact/collision exposure, such as number of games or cumulative biomechanical forces. What is clear is that the decision to retire will be highly individualized, and it should be based on a thorough clinical assessment. Because the symptoms for chronic impairment after repeated concussions are nonspecific, objective evidence should be obtained and alternative diagnoses that would explain the athletes' symptoms should be considered, particularly alternative diagnoses that are treatable (Table 22-2). Health care providers should use all the clinical tools available, including history, neurologic examination, comprehensive neuropsychometric testing, and neuroimaging. However, the decision to retire from sport due to neurological decline should be made by or in consultation with a neurologist, who can provide input on the specific examination findings.

Table 22-2

Differential Diagnosis for Chronic Postconcussive Symptoms

Primary headache disorders (migraine, tension-type headache)
Secondary headache disorders (posttraumatic headache, cervicogenic headache, spontaneous intracranial hypotension, cerebral venous sinus thrombosis)
Learning disabilities (attention deficit disorder, dyslexia)
Psychiatric illnesses (depression, anxiety, posttraumatic stress disorder)
Primary sleep disorders (insomnia, hypersomnia)
Autonomic disorders (postural orthostatic tachycardia syndrome, orthostatic hypotension)
Seizure disorders
Chronic pain disorders, chronic fatigue syndrome, fibromyalgia
Other systemic disorders (anemia, hypo-/hyperthyroidism, autoimmune disorders, vitamin D or B_{12} deficiencies)

References

1. Savica R, Parisi JE, Wold LE, Josephs KA, Ahlskog JE. High school football and risk of neuro-degeneration: a community-based study. *Mayo Clin Proc*. 2012;87(4):335-340.
2. Lehman EJ, Hein MJ, Baron SL, Gersic CM. Neurodegenerative causes of death among retired National Football League players. *Neurology*. 2012;79(19):1970-1974.
3. Guskiewicz KM, Marshall SW, Bailes J, et al. Association between recurrent concussion and late-life cognitive impairment in retired professional football players. *Neurosurgery*. 2005;57(4):719-726.
4. Kutner KC, Erlanger DM, Tsai J, Jordan B, Relkin NR. Lower cognitive performance of older football players possessing apolipoprotein E epsilon 4. *Neurosurgery*. 2000;47(3):651-657.
5. Matser JT, Kessels AG, Lezak MD, Troost J. A dose-response relation of headers and concussions with cognitive impairment in professional soccer players. *J Clin Exp Neuropsychol*. 2001;23(6):770-774.
6. Wall SE, Williams WH, Cartwright-Hatton S, et al. Neuropsychological dysfunction following repeat concussions in jockeys. *J Neurol Neurosurg Psychiatry*. 2006;77(4):518-520.
7. Giza CC, Kutcher JS, Ashwal S, et al. Summary of evidence-based guideline update: evaluation and management of concussion in sports: report of the Guideline Development Subcommittee of the American Academy of Neurology. *Neurology*. 2013;80(24):2250-2257.
8. Guskiewicz KM, Marshall SW, Bailes J, et al. Recurrent concussion and risk of depression in retired professional football players. *Med Sci Sports Exerc*. 2007;39(6):903-909.
9. Kerr ZY, Marshall SW, Harding HP Jr, Guskiewicz KM. Nine-year risk of depression diagnosis increases with increasing self-reported concussions in retired professional football players. *Am J Sports Med*. 2012;40(10):2206-2212.
10. Vargas BB, Dodick DW. Posttraumatic headache. *Curr Opin Neurol*. 2012;25(3):284-289.
11. Eisenberg MA, Andrea J, Meehan W, Mannix R. Time interval between concussions and symptom duration. *Pediatrics*. 2013;132(1):8-17.
12. Guskiewicz KM, McCrea M, Marshall SW, et al. Cumulative effects associated with recurrent concussion in collegiate football players: the NCAA Concussion Study. *JAMA*. 2003;290(19):2549-2555.

WHAT ARE THE LONG-TERM CONCERNS WITH CONCUSSION?

Steven P. Broglio, PhD, ATC and Douglas Martini, MS

Researchers have been questioning and evaluating the long-term effects of concussion for several years. Early investigations typically implemented standard clinical assessments (eg, neurocognitive tests) in young adult athletes. In general, the findings from these studies indicated there were no significant differences between those with and without an injury. In one of these studies, the authors speculated that concussion did not have an effect on cognitive health beyond the acute stage of injury *or* the tools being used at the time were not sensitive to the subtle changes being brought about by injury.[1] To date, the former is looking less and less likely and the latter more and more feasible.

The return to preinjury levels of functioning from concussion is thought to occur within 2 weeks in adults. This notion has been derived from the implementation of clinical tests in concussed athletes that evaluate concussion-related symptoms, postural control, and neurocognitive function. Although each of these tests is highly capable of evaluating gross declines following injury, they do not appear to be sensitive to subtle declines that persist for years after injury. For example, one

Valovich McLeod TC, ed. *Quick Questions in Sport-Related Concussion: Expert Advice in Sports Medicine* (pp 119-121). © 2015 Taylor & Francis Group.

investigation enrolled young adults with and without a concussion history. Those with a concussion history were, on average, 3.2 years postinjury. All participants completed a computer-based neurocognitive assessment that is commonly used for concussion management and the visual oddball task while event-related potentials (ERPs) (ie, cerebral activity) were being recorded. Similar to previous works, the results indicated no difference between the 2 groups on the neurocognitive evaluation. Surprisingly, the ERP evaluation indicated those with a concussion history showed lowered cerebral activation in relation to attentional resources and a decreased ability to suppress errant responses. Although these subtle changes were present in the concussion history group, they were not of the magnitude that changed the daily functioning of the participants.[2]

Second to this investigation was a study evaluating the effects of concussion on postural control. Athletes with a concussion history were, on average, 2.9 years postinjury, while a group of nonconcussed athletes served as controls. The preseason postural control evaluation yielded no differences in common balance measures, but subtle differences were noted between the 2 groups when their sway patterns were evaluated. That is, the concussed group showed a decline in the complexity of their mediolateral (ML) sway, suggesting that the nonconcussed group had more control of their ML movements.[3] These changes parallel postural control declines reported in healthy older adults but also suggest that without intervention, those with a concussion history may be more susceptible to falls and further injury later in life.

A follow-up to the postural control investigation evaluated for changes in gait in young adults with and without a concussion history. In this study, the concussed group was 6 years postinjury. Each participant was evaluated on 4 gait conditions: with and without a brief cognitive task and/or stepping over an obstacle. The cognitive task was also completed while seated, but similar to other studies implementing cognitive tests, there were no differences between the 2 groups under any conditions. Gait variables that are typically evaluated (eg, speed, stance length, and width) did not differ between groups either. What did differ was the time spent in single-leg stance (ie, swing phase) and the time in double-leg stance. For these measures, the previously concussed group showed greater time in double-leg stance and less time in single-leg stance than the healthy participants. When viewed in conjunction with the balance findings above, the authors felt the previously concussed participants had adopted a more conservative and safer gait pattern to protect themselves from falls.[4] Similar to the study on balance, this gait pattern is common among older adults who are otherwise injury free.

These study findings do not directly indicate that sustaining one or more concussions will result in cognitive function or motor control (ie, gait and balance) declines to a degree that will have a meaningful influence later in life. But if they do, the literature cited here suggests that concussion can no longer be thought of as a transient injury void of long-term consequences. However, caution is warranted. One cannot assume that just because an athlete sustains a concussion during high school, he or she is now predisposed to significant late-life cognitive decline. Indeed, research indicating that multiple concussions may result in higher rates of depression and mild cognitive impairment[5,6] was conducted on professional athletes with years of exposure to subconcussive impacts and numerous unreported concussions. This is not the same level of exposure for the average individual.

However, even if the concussion sets the wheels in motion for decline, numerous factors will play a role. For example, the individual's genetic profile, family history of cognitive issues, exercise, and alcohol consumption, along with other factors, may influence cognitive change in a positive or negative manner over time.[7] Importantly, the majority of individuals who sustain concussions during athletic events end their careers with high school, which appears to have no relation to later life changes.[8] This is in contrast to highly publicized reports of professional athletes with decades of exposure to head impacts and concussions.

References

1. Broglio SP, Ferrara MS, Piland SG, Anderson RB. Concussion history is not a predictor of computerized neurocognitive performance. *Br J Sports Med.* 2006;40(9):802-805.
2. Broglio SP, Pontifex MB, O'Connor P, Hillman CH. The persistent effects of concussion on neuroelectric indices of attention. *J Neurotrauma.* 2009;26(9):1463-1470.
3. Sosnoff JJ, Broglio SP, Shin S, Ferrara MS. Previous mild traumatic brain injury and postural control dynamics. *J Athl Train.* 2011;46(1):85-91.
4. Martini DN, Sabin MJ, DePesa SA, et al. The chronic effects of concussion on gait. *Arch Phys Med Rehabil.* 2011;92(4):585-589.
5. Guskiewicz KM, Marshall SW, Bailes J, et al. Recurrent concussion and risk of depression in retired professional football players. *Med Sci Sports Exerc.* 2007;39(6):903-909.
6. Guskiewicz KM, Marshall SW, Bailes J, et al. Association between recurrent concussion and late-life cognitive impairment in retired professional football players. *Neurosurgery.* 2005;57(4):719-726.
7. Broglio SP, Eckner JT, Paulson H, Kutcher JS. Cognitive decline and aging: the role of concussive and sub-concussive impacts. *Exerc Sport Sci Rev.* 2012;40(3):138-144.
8. Savica R, Parisi JE, Wold LE, Josephs KA, Ahlskog JE. High school football and risk of neurodegeneration: a community-based study. *Mayo Clin Proc.* 2012;87(4):335-340.

HOW CAN WE PREDICT IF A PATIENT WILL HAVE A PROTRACTED RECOVERY FOLLOWING CONCUSSION?

Ian A. McLeod, PA-C, ATC

Having 15-plus years of experience working with athletes, I have found that the question that I am almost always asked after informing an athlete of the nature and severity of his or her injury is, "How long will I be out?" For the most part, I am able to provide an estimated time frame with some degree of certainty, unless the athlete has sustained a concussion, because in those cases there is some degree of uncertainty. The reason for the uncertainty is that, unlike for most musculoskeletal injuries, the severity of a concussion based on initial examination findings cannot be graded by clinicians. Not knowing the severity of the injury limits our ability to predict the time frame for recovery. What we do know is that 80% to 90% of adults who sustain a concussion will recover within 7 to 10 days and that children may have a longer time frame for recovery.[1] Athletes who do not recover within this time frame are considered to have a protracted recovery. Because there is value in identifying which athletes may have a protracted recovery sooner rather than later, it is important that clinicians be aware of information that is available to help predict if an athlete will have a protracted recovery. The value in identifying these

Valovich McLeod TC, ed. *Quick Questions in Sport-Related Concussion: Expert Advice in Sports Medicine* (pp 123-127).
© 2015 Taylor & Francis Group.

individuals early in the recovery process is that they will benefit greatly from work or school accommodations and management by a multidisciplinary team of health care providers who specialize in the management of sport-related concussion.[1]

Identifying Risk Factors Prior to Injury

Several risk factors have been identified that may indicate that a patient may have a prolonged recovery even prior to a concussion. These include concussion history, age, sex, and the presence of comorbid conditions, such as attention deficit disorder, learning disabilities, mood disorders, and migraine headaches. Although the evidence is not conclusive that these factors always lead to a prolonged recovery, it is important for clinicians to note any of these factors during the preparticipation examination for management of any subsequent concussion sustained by the patient. Furthermore, these, along with other intrinsic and extrinsic factors, have been identified as concussion-modifying factors, with suggestions to treat patients with these conditions in a more conservative manner.[1]

Patients with a *history of prior concussions* may have a protracted recovery with subsequent injuries.[2,3] There is speculation that with each concussion, the threshold to sustain a concussion lowers and injuries may occur with lesser impacts. In addition, the time between concussive injuries is important, with evidence that concussions that occur in closer proximity to each other result in a longer recovery.[1] Therefore, clinicians should solicit a good concussion history with each concussion evaluation and educate patients that they may take longer to recover because of their prior concussions.

Age has also been identified as a possible risk factor resulting in a protracted recovery. Due to the anatomical differences between children and adults, such as weaker neck musculature and larger head-to-neck ratio, there is concern that the impacts that result in concussion may result in a more severe clinical presentation of concussion. This may lead to a longer recovery, as noted by studies that have found that both symptom and neurocognitive recovery takes longer in children than in adults.[3,4]

Sex may also play a role in determining protracted recovery. Females tend to report more concussion-related symptoms and deficits in neurocognitive function following injury, which may lead to a longer recovery.[1,3,4] Because the presence of symptoms may suggest a protracted recovery, it is important for clinicians to obtain a thorough symptom report, via symptom scale or inventory, during each visit with the patient.

Other *comorbid conditions* may also increase the risk of a prolonged recovery following concussion. Patients with a medical history that includes attention deficit disorder, learning disabilities, or mood disorders, such as anxiety and depression, may have a protracted recovery.[4] Clinicians will need to consider the symptom severity prior to the concussion and aim to identify if the postinjury symptoms are the result of the concussion or the underlying condition. Stronger evidence exists that patients with a migraine headache history may present with a greater number of symptoms, greater neurocognitive impairments, and take longer to recover after a concussion.[4]

Predictors Following Concussion

Although information gained from the patient's past medical history can help identify patients who might be at risk for a protracted recovery prior to an injury occurring, several postinjury characteristics may also help clinicians identify patients who may be at risk for a longer recovery. These include the initial overall symptom presentation, presence of specific symptoms, and immediate cognitive deficits.[2-5]

The nature, duration, and severity of the symptoms present at the time of injury may be important predictors of prolonged recovery.[2,3] In a review of prolonged recovery factors, Makdissi et al[2] suggest that in studies of American and Australian football, higher numbers of reported symptoms and higher severity score of those symptoms are positively correlated to recovery time. More specifically, athletes who report at least 4 symptoms at the time of injury tend to have a prolonged recovery.[2] Therefore, it is important for health care providers assessing the concussion at the time of injury to inquire about a broad range of symptoms, ideally using a symptom inventory. Clinicians who are evaluating a patient in the office should ask questions specific to the *current* symptoms the patient is experiencing and ask about the type, nature, and duration of symptoms present *immediately after the injury*.

In addition to the general symptom presentation that may predict a protracted recovery, the presence of specific symptoms during the initial evaluation may also be of concern. Loss of consciousness for greater than 1 minute, retrograde and anterograde posttraumatic amnesia, fatigue, prolonged headache, and fogginess have all been identified as predictors.[4] Cognitive symptoms such as confusion, memory problems, and deficits in the cognitive functions of visual memory and processing speed have also been associated with delayed resolution of symptoms leading to a prolonged recovery.[4] Although more research needs to be done in this area, one prognostic study[5] identified that computerized reaction time scores and the presence of migraine-like symptoms (Table 24-1) were predictive of protracted recovery.

Clinicians who evaluate patients following concussion should pay special consideration to risk factors for and prognostic indicators of a protracted recovery. Age, sex, prior concussion history, comorbid conditions, immediate symptom

Table 24-1
Migraine Symptom Classification

Headache	Sensitivity to light
Nausea	Sensitivity to noise
Vomiting	Numbness or tingling
Balance problems	Visual problems
Dizziness	

Table 24-2
Outcome Measures That May Assist Clinicians With Patients Having a Protracted Recovery[3]

Domain	Questionnaire/Assessment Tool
Anxiety and depression	Hospital Anxiety and Depression Scale
	Beck Depression Inventory
	Depression Anxiety Stress Scale
	Profile of Mood States
Headache and migraine	Headache Impact Test
	Migraine Disability Assessment
General health and disability	Short Form 36
	Health Survey Questionnaire
Sleep	Medical Outcomes Study Sleep Scale Survey
Drug and alcohol use	Drug Abuse Screening Test
	Alcohol Disorders Identification Test

presentation, and acute cognitive dysfunction should raise your suspicion that a patient may have a prolonged recovery. In those cases, the management plan may then require the inclusion of more detailed history and screening (Table 24-2) and additional specialists to manage the injury. Prompt identification of athletes at risk for prolonged recovery will allow for early initiation of interventions that can assist with creating the optimal environment for the recovery process (eg, physical therapy for vestibular rehabilitation, work and/or school accommodations, neuropsychology referral). Clinicians who have a firm understanding of the risk factors and prognostic indicators for prolonged recovery will find that they are better prepared to educate athletes, parents, and coaches regarding the potential severity of an injury and, in turn, the projected time frame for recovery.

References

1. McCrory P, Meeuwisse WH, Aubry M, et al. Consensus statement on concussion in sport: the 4th International Conference on Concussion in Sport held in Zurich, November 2012. *Br J Sports Med*. 2013;47(5):250-258.
2. Makdissi M, Cantu RC, Johnston KM, McCrory P, Meeuwisse WH. The difficult concussion patient: what is the best approach to investigation and management of persistent (> 10 days) postconcussive symptoms? *Br J Sports Med*. 2013;47(5):308-313.
3. Giza CC, Kutcher JS, Ashwal S, et al. Summary of evidence-based guideline update: evaluation and management of concussion in sports: report of the Guideline Development Subcommittee of the American Academy of Neurology. *Neurology*. 2013;80(24):2250-2257.
4. Scopaz KA, Hatzenbuehler JR. Risk modifiers for concussion and prolonged recovery. *Sports Health*. 2013;5(6):537-541.
5. Lau B, Lovell MR, Collins MW, Pardini J. Neurocognitive and symptom predictors of recovery in high school athletes. *Clin J Sport Med*. 2009;19(3):216-221.

DO SUBCONCUSSIVE BLOWS PLACE ATHLETES AT JUST AS MUCH RISK FOR FUTURE NEGATIVE SEQUELAE AS ATHLETES WITH DIAGNOSED CONCUSSIONS?

Steven P. Broglio, PhD, ATC and Douglas Martini, MS

The long-term consequences of subconcussive impacts (ie, impacts to the head that do not result in a concussion) are fundamentally unknown. Chronic traumatic encephalopathy (CTE) has been described as a progressive neurodegenerative disease resulting from repeated concussive and subconcussive head impacts. In short, it is believed that repeated exposure to head impacts results in a hyper-phosphorylization of tau proteins, which compromises microtubule structure. The hyperphosphorylized proteins are believed to aggregate in the surrounding tissue and form tau fibrils or neurofibrillary tangles, but the actual mechanisms are still unknown. CTE has been reported primarily in former elite athletes who have sustained decades of head impacts, as well as numerous diagnosed and undiagnosed concussions. Elite athletes are a relatively small and unique population, and they have sustained decades of head impacts during their high school, collegiate, and professional careers. Conversely, over 1 million athletes participate in high school football each year and have a relatively short athletic career. As such, elite-level athletes sustain a far greater number of concussive and subconcussive impacts across their football career relative to the average athlete who is done playing organized

Valovich McLeod TC, ed. *Quick Questions in Sport-Related
Concussion: Expert Advice in Sports Medicine* (pp 129-131).
© 2015 Taylor & Francis Group.

football after high school. Unfortunately, the elite cases receive the most attention due to media coverage and a general lack of understanding resulting from the scientific unknowns.

Despite this, one cannot assume that repeated blows to the head, in absence of concussion, are void of consequences. For example, one group of investigators evaluated high school football athletes preseason on a standard computer-based cognitive assessment and cerebral imaging using functional magnetic resonance imaging (fMRI). During the season, each athlete had his or her head impacts monitored for frequency, location, and magnitude (ie, postimpact accelerations) and were readministered the baseline tests at random intervals. The authors reported that no athlete sustained a concussion or showed a measurable decline on the computerized neurocognitive assessment. However, they did demonstrate significant changes on the fMRI scans that correlated positively with head impact frequency. That is, greater fMRI changes were associated with a high number of impacts.[1] What remains unknown is whether the athletes return to their preseason levels of functioning or if the changes are permanent.

Based on this finding, it is feasible for there to be 3 populations of individuals when considering the chronic effects of concussions and/or subconcussive impacts. There is the control population, or group of individuals with no previous concussion and few subconcussive impacts. This population either never played sports or never participated in contact/collision sports, and any head impacts were the result of routine living. A second group may have suffered a couple of concussions and/or many subconcussive impacts. This group likely participated in contact/collision sports up to and possibly through college, though most of this population ended their athletic career with high school graduation. Finally, the third and most extreme population are those who played professionally and/or sustained a substantial number of concussions/subconcussive impacts. This is the smallest population but the one that gets the most coverage in that most of what is known about the chronic effects is from individuals in this population. How these groups are differentiated from each other is entirely unknown. The current literature cannot definitively identify a specific number of concussions and/or subconcussive impacts that would place someone into one of these 3 groups, but one could imagine that certain athletes would fall into the different categories.

Ultimately, to say that a single concussion or a small number of subconcussive impacts will cause chronic changes in an individual's life is likely a gross overstatement. Up to 3.8 million concussions result from sport and recreation each year. These injuries are largely in the younger population, yet a significant number of these individuals do not complain about poor cognitive health later in life. In addition, there are former professional-level football athletes with and without documented concussions who are cognitively no different from their peers who did not play football. Conversely, one investigator reported the presence of CTE in a collegiate athlete who had no documented concussions.[2] If and how this pathology affected his daily life is unknown. Believing that there is a causal relationship between concussions and/or subconcussive impacts is incorrect. Just as there is no known impact threshold value for sustaining a concussion, so too is there no known threshold for concussive/subconcussive impacts leading to late-life impairments.

In the final analysis, it is feasible that repeated exposure to concussive and subconcussive forces can bring about long-term cognitive decline. The frequency, magnitude, or combination of both that will bring about this decline, however, is unknown. Regardless, sporting organizations and conferences have begun limiting contact practices in an effort to reduce exposure, but there is no evidence this will have an effect on cognitive functioning decades after the fact. Indeed, there is little research evaluating the relationship between contact and noncontact practices and head impacts.[3,4]

References

1. Talavage TM, Nauman E, Breedlove EL, et al. Functionally-detected cognitive impairment in high school football players without clinically diagnosed concussion. *J Neurotrauma.* 2014;31(4):327-338.
2. McKee AC, Stein TD, Nowinski CJ, et al. The spectrum of disease in chronic traumatic encephalopathy. *Brain.* 2012;136(Pt1):43-64.
3. Mihalik JP, Bell DR, Marshall SW, Guskiewicz KM. Measurement of head impacts in collegiate football players: an investigation of positional and event-type differences. *Neurosurgery.* 2007;61(6):1229-1235.
4. Broglio SP, Martini DN, Kasper L, Eckner JT, Kutcher JS. Estimation of head impact exposure in high school football: implications for regulating contact practices. *Am J Sports Med.* 2013;41(12):2877-2884.

HOW SHOULD I MANAGE CONCUSSION IN ATHLETES WITH LEARNING DISABILITIES, EPILEPSY, DEPRESSION, OR ANXIETY?

Javier Cárdenas, MD and
Tamara C. Valovich McLeod, PhD, ATC, FNATA

Managing concussion in patients with medical conditions can be a challenging endeavor, largely due to exacerbation of the underlying condition. Many of these underlying conditions are included as concussion modifiers that may influence recovery after a concussion and should therefore warrant a more conservative approach to management.[1] Clinicians need to attempt to identify which symptoms preceded the concussion, which symptoms resulted from the concussion, and which symptoms worsened after the concussion.[2] For example, individuals with migraine who sustain a concussion tend to have more migraines and migraine-like symptoms that are difficult to tease out from possible symptoms of a concussive injury. Those with learning disabilities who sustain a concussion tend to have greater trouble in school, just as those with depression and anxiety tend to have more sadness and anxiety following the concussion. In addition to magnifying symptoms, these underlying conditions may prolong the typical course of recovery.[3] Therefore, appropriate management of patients with underlying medical conditions should

Valovich McLeod TC, ed. *Quick Questions in Sport-Related Concussion: Expert Advice in Sports Medicine* (pp 133-135).
© 2015 Taylor & Francis Group.

begin during the preparticipation examination and include a more thorough history following a concussion to provide an individualized management plan in these populations.

Learning disabilities in the adolescent and student-athlete population are incredibly common due to greater efforts in identification and management through academic accommodations. Athletes with learning disabilities pose a unique set of challenges in concussion management, particularly in an age of widespread use of computerized cognitive testing. Learning disabilities may include problems with memory, concentration, and attention—several cognitive domains that are affected by and overlap with symptoms of a concussion.

Normative data for this population are limited; therefore, baseline testing in this population is particularly important if cognitive evaluations are to be used in postinjury assessment and management of concussion. Furthermore, identifying not only the learning disability but also any prior concussions is imperative, as one study reported that college athletes with a learning disability and history of prior concussion reported lower baseline cognitive functioning.[4] Clinicians will also need to decide whether patients being managed with a specific prescription should take the baseline cognitive test while on or off the medication.

Because of the varied nature of learning disabilities, one can expect a variety of cognitive deficits after a concussion. For example, students with a learning disability in language may have greater difficulty with reading and writing. Those with attention deficit hyperactivity disorder are likely to have greater challenges with impulse control and focus. The assistance of a neuropsychologist is particularly helpful in managing concussion in student athletes before and after a concussion. After a concussion, athletes with learning disabilities should receive academic accommodations tailored to their needs. These may include preferential seating, additional time for assignments or tests, and a reduction in homework volume.

Although children and adolescents with epilepsy should not be prohibited from athletics, an understanding of seizures in head trauma is important to medical management. An immediate (within 5 minutes) posttraumatic seizure in the setting of a head injury is not uncommon and does not confer a greater risk of epilepsy in the future. This is in contrast to seizures that occur early (greater than 5 minutes but less than 7 days) or late (greater than 7 days) after a more severe head injury.[5] The risk of epilepsy in the general population is approximately 1%, while concussion increases that risk up to 4%. Athletes with a known history of epilepsy are more likely to have a seizure immediately after a concussion and any time thereafter, depending on their preinjury seizure burden. Seizures are considered a red flag in the setting of a concussion and should be evaluated immediately by a health care provider. Often, patients with epilepsy will require an increase in their antiepileptic medication because of increased seizure activity following a concussion. However, practitioners should recognize that doing so may also cause fatigue and cognitive side effects.

According to the National Institute for Mental Health, the incidence of depression in adolescence is approximately 11%.[6] Behavioral symptoms after a concussion include irritability, depression, anxiety, and emotional instability. As such, exacerbation of behavioral symptoms in depressed youth after a concussion is common. Screening for anxiety, depression, and suicidal tendencies is a requisite in obtaining a past medical history and for assessing ongoing symptoms. This may include the use of screening tools such as the Patient Health Questionnaire (PHQ-9) or the Generalized Anxiety Disorder 7-item scale. Psychologists, psychiatrists, and specialists trained in adolescent medicine should be included in the care of athletes who exhibit prolonged or severe behavioral symptoms after a concussion. Care should be taken in understanding the behavioral side effects of prescribed medication and considerations made for initiating antidepressants in this population.

Regardless of the underlying medical condition, clinicians need to have a heightened awareness for the effects of concussion in these patients. Ideally, this begins with a thorough preparticipation examination to better characterize the type, frequency, and duration of symptoms related to the condition. In addition, preseason baseline scores, including an assessment of symptoms, cognitive function, and postural control are obtained. Clinicians should also include other providers with expertise in the condition as members of the concussion management team to assist in the follow-up care of a concussed patient. Lastly, the return-to-play criteria may need to be modified to account for preinjury prescription medications, prior concussion history, and the time to symptom resolution, which may result in a more conservative approach and longer progression prior to full clearance to participate.

References

1. McCrory P, Meeuwisse WH, Aubry M, et al. Consensus statement on concussion in sport: the 4th International Conference on Concussion in Sport held in Zurich, November 2012. *Br J Sports Med.* 2013;47(5):250-258.
2. Harmon KG, Drezner J, Gammons M, et al. American Medical Society for Sports Medicine position statement: concussion in sport. *Clin J Sport Med.* 2013;23(1):1-18.
3. Makdissi M, Cantu RC, Johnston KM, McCrory P, Meeuwisse WH. The difficult concussion patient: what is the best approach to investigation and management of persistent (> 10 days) postconcussive symptoms? *Br J Sports Med.* 2013;47(5):308-313.
4. Collins MW, Grindel SH, Lovell MR, et al. Relationship between concussion and neuropsychological performance in college football players. *JAMA.* 1999;282(10):964-970.
5. Lowenstein DH. Epilepsy after head injury: an overview. *Epilepsia.* 2009;50 Suppl 2:4-9.
6. Kessler RC. *National Comorbidity Survey: Adolescent Supplement (NCS-A), 2001-2004. ICPSR28581-v5:* Inter-university Consortium for Political and Social Research; 2013.

ARE THERE ANY MEDICATIONS THAT MAY BE USEFUL IN THE MANAGEMENT OF CONCUSSIONS?

Javier Cárdenas, MD and
Tamara C. Valovich McLeod, PhD, ATC, FNATA

Administration of medications, as in any other disease or illness, should be done with great deliberation. Most concussions exhibit a natural course of immediate symptom presentation followed by steady improvement and resolution within days to weeks. In the vast majority of cases, medication is unnecessary. However, symptomatic treatment of physical, behavioral, and cognitive disturbances with medication is sometimes necessary, particularly when prolonged or severe symptoms exist (Table 27-1).[1,2]

The prescription of any pharmacological agent should be considered after a period of conservative treatment and with a goal of reducing or managing specific symptoms.[1-3] The decision to use pharmacological agents usually occurs if a patient has symptoms lasting longer than the typical recovery period and when these symptoms significantly impact the patient's quality of life.[2] Clinicians should understand that no pharmacological interventions have been shown to speed recovery following concussion or prevent secondary brain injury.[4] Furthermore, it

Valovich McLeod TC, ed. *Quick Questions in Sport-Related Concussion: Expert Advice in Sports Medicine* (pp 137-140).
© 2015 Taylor & Francis Group.

Table 27-1

Medications for Concussion-Related Symptoms

Symptom	Medication Class	Medications
Somatic: headache	Analgesics	Acetaminophen
	Nonsteroidal anti-inflammatory drugs	Ibuprofen, naproxen, diclofenac
	Antidepressants	Amitriptyline, nortriptyline
	Anticonvulsants	Valproic acid, topiramate, gabapentin
	Beta-adrenergic antagonists	Propranolol, metoprolol
Somatic: dizziness	Vestibular suppressants	Meclizine, scopolamine
	Benzodiazepines	Lorazepam, clonazepam, diazepam
Somatic: fatigue	Neurostimulants	Methylphenidate, destroamphetamine, modafinil, amantadine
Somatic: nausea	Antiemetics	Ondansetron, promethazine
Sleep disturbances	Sedative-hypnotics	Zolpidem
	Serotonin modulators	Trazodone
	Alpha-adrenergic antagonists	Prazosin
	Supplement	Melatonin
Emotional: depression	Tricyclic antidepressants	Amitriptyline, nortriptyline
	Selective serotonin reuptake inhibitors (SSRIs)	Sertraline, citalopram, escitalopram, paroxetine, fluoxetine
Emotional: anxiety	Benzodiazepines	Lorazepam, clonazepam, diazepam
Cognitive	Neurostimulants	Methylphenidate, dextroamphetamine, modafinil, amantadine, atomoxetine
	SSRIs	Sertraline, fluoxetine
	Acetylcholinesterase inhibitors	Donepezil, rivastigmine, galantamine

Adapted from Petraglia AL, Maroon JC, Bailes JE. From the field of play to the field of combat: a review of the pharmacological management of concussion. *Neurosurgery.* 2012;70(6):1520-1533.

is important to understand the concerns with pharmacological therapy, including masking concussion-related symptoms, additional symptoms resulting from side effects of medications, and difficulty with interpretation of neurological and cognitive assessments due to medication use.[1,4]

Headache, the most common physical symptom after a concussion, is typically treated with over-the-counter analgesics. Acetaminophen is preferred within the first 72 hours, as the risk of intracranial hemorrhage is greatest in this period of time. Nonsteroidal anti-inflammatory drugs (NSAIDs) and aspirin are generally not recommended during the acute period after injury because of the risk of hemorrhage. Rebound headaches are a common consequence of analgesic overuse that often extend physical symptoms and can make it difficult to determine the course of recovery.[5] In these cases, the use of headache-prevention medications, such as amitriptyline, should be considered. Such medications do not cause rebound headaches and may provide symptomatic relief to ailing patients. Headache-prevention medications have other primary uses, including antidepressants, anticonvulsants, and antihypertensives. The side-effect profile can also be useful in determining the most appropriate medication for headache prevention. Administration of these medications is best made in consultation with a specialist in headaches.

Insomnia and other sleep disturbances after a concussion typically follow an initial period of hypersomnia. Lack of sleep commonly exacerbates other postconcussive symptoms, including headaches, daytime fatigue, and impaired cognition. Treatment of insomnia can provide relief of multiple symptoms and accelerate overall recovery. However, sleep aids may not always provide restful sleep and have their own set of side effects, which can include dizziness, lightheadedness, headache, and daytime drowsiness. In many instances, the treatment of other symptoms, such as headaches, with medications such as antidepressants or anticonvulsants that cause fatigue may provide relief to multiple symptoms, especially when used with good sleep hygiene techniques.

Treatment of depression and anxiety with antidepressants and anxiolytics, respectively, should be done in consultation with a mental health provider. Medical treatment is best when combined with behavioral-cognitive therapy. Those being treated for anxiety or depression and on medication may require a temporary increase in dosage while recovering from injury.

Medical treatment for cognitive deficits is typically unnecessary, although a body of literature is developing to address this issue. Stimulant medication is utilized in those with a known history of attention deficit hyperactivity disorder (ADHD) and sometimes increased if the athlete is already taking a medication for this condition. Medications typically reserved for those with moderate or severe traumatic brain injury, such as the off-label use of amantadine, are being studied but are not a standard of care. One small retrospective study reported that adolescents with a prolonged recovery of more than 21 days noted improvements in verbal memory and reaction time and a decrease in symptoms when treated with 100 mg of amantadine twice daily for 3 to 4 weeks.[6]

One important consideration with medication use following sport-related concussion is related to returning the patient to activity. Recommendations state that patients should be free of all symptoms and return to near baseline on adjunct assessments of cognition and balance prior to considering a return-to-play progression.[1,3] These recommendations hold true for patients who were prescribed medications postconcussion but also include the caveat that all pharmacological agents be discontinued prior to beginning a return-to-play progression.

References

1. Harmon KG, Drezner J, Gammons M, et al. American Medical Society for Sports Medicine position statement: concussion in sport. *Clin J Sport Med*. 2013;23(1):1-18.
2. Meehan WP. Medical therapies for concussion. *Clin Sports Med*. 2011;30(1):115-124.
3. McCrory P, Meeuwisse WH, Aubry M, et al. Consensus statement on concussion in sport: the 4th International Conference on Concussion in Sport held in Zurich, November 2012. *Br J Sports Med*. 2013;47(5):250-258.
4. Beauchamp K, Mutlak H, Smith WR, Shohami E, Stahel PF. Pharmacology of traumatic brain injury: where is the "golden bullet"? *Mol Med*. 2008;14(11-12):731-740.
5. Petraglia AL, Maroon JC, Bailes JE. From the field of play to the field of combat: a review of the pharmacological management of concussion. *Neurosurgery*. 2012;70(6):1520-1533.
6. Reddy CC, Collins M, Lovell M, Kontos AP. Efficacy of amantadine treatment on symptoms and neurocognitive performance among adolescents following sports-related concussion. *J Head Trauma Rehabil*. 2013;28(4):260-265.

ARE THERE ANY REHABILITATION EXERCISES THAT HELP A CONCUSSED ATHLETE HEAL FASTER?

Johna K. Register-Mihalik, PhD, LAT, ATC and
Jason P. Mihalik, PhD, CAT(C), ATC

Although rehabilitation is an integral component for the treatment of traumatic brain injury (TBI) patients, it is still the most misunderstood component of an already complex injury, specifically in those who suffer a concussion. The majority of patients suffering from concussion typically recover within 2 to 3 weeks and may not appear to initially require a rehabilitation period. However, new directives and discussion in our field of concussion management are encouraging clinicians to take a more active management approach following the initial rest period postconcussion. These include helping patients to set short- and long-term goals as they would with any other sport-related musculoskeletal injury, and to begin supervised and controlled integration into activities of daily living as well as monitored light physical activities. In addition, rehabilitation exercises may be most beneficial to individuals who do not recover in a typical time frame and experience prolonged concussion symptoms (eg, longer than 3 weeks). All of these activities should be considered in the context of the individual patient and monitored for symptom exacerbation

Valovich McLeod TC, ed. *Quick Questions in Sport-Related Concussion: Expert Advice in Sports Medicine* (pp 141-143).
© 2015 Taylor & Francis Group.

because symptom exacerbation during low-intensity activities may be an indicator of ongoing dysfunction. In guiding active approaches to treatment, the ongoing neurometabolic demands that occur postconcussion need to be initially managed, not allowing the physiological thresholds associated with activity to be exceeded.[1]

Few studies investigating activity levels following concussion are available. Although retrospective, one of the only studies to look at activity levels following concussion found that individuals with the least and those with the most physical and cognitive activity had the worst outcomes. This same study found that those patients who reported participating in low-intensity (nonsport) activities following injury were the least impaired during clinical follow-up. We note, of course, that all patients in the study experienced declines relative to preseason baseline testing regardless of activity level. This study suggests monitored low-intensity activities may potentially aid the concussion-recovery process. There is evidence to suggest that a graduated exercise treadmill program, using heart rate as a reference, may help to improve symptoms in individuals with persistent concussive symptoms.[2] Vestibular rehabilitation is believed to benefit those individuals who continue to display vestibular deficits following concussion; these rehabilitation exercises were shown to improve dizziness, gait, and balance dysfunction.[3] The most commonly prescribed vestibular exercises include eye-head coordination exercises, static balance tasks, and ambulation exercises.[4]

The aforementioned studies are limited by small sample sizes. Additionally, there is a paucity of literature with respect to rehabilitation protocols specific to concussion. Notwithstanding, the TBI literature may provide us with unique insights into rehabilitation strategies clinicians may employ with concussion patients experiencing persistent issues. Typical therapy protocols for TBI—namely moderate-to-severe TBI—involve an interdisciplinary approach combining the efforts of athletic trainers, physical therapists, speech therapists, occupational therapists, and/or neuropsychologists.[5] Reported advantages to rehabilitation approaches include increased patient motivation and acceptance of treatment and an increase in the patients' ability to generalize and transfer treatment gains from treatment settings to their ultimate return goal. Although little evidence exists, use of divided-attention tasks in the rehabilitation process has also been discussed. These activities include those where more than one attentional activity (eg, a balance/motor activity) is paired with a cognitive activity, and the two are performed at the same time.

The underlying premise of divided-attention tasks—sometimes referred to as dual tasking—is that the inclusion of combined activities allows the clinician to more realistically challenge the patient in an environment that approximates activities of daily living and, in more advanced stages of rehabilitation, sport-specific activities. For example, clinical testing paradigms that include neurocognitive and balance testing perform these evaluations in isolation. Realistically, however,

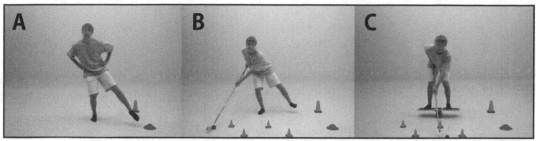

Figure 28-1. Sample dual-task exercise progression. (A) Patient performs single-leg stance and is instructed to reach out to the circular marker when clinician says an odd number and reach for the pylon when clinician says an even number. (B) The addition of sport-specific activity of stickhandling the ball around the cones while performing the same task as described in A. (C) Patient balance activities intensify while performing sport-specific stickhandling activity. Athlete is asked to perform serial sevens (reciting numbers in reverse order beginning with 100...93...86...etc) while maintaining balance and stickhandling speed.

patient-athletes must function cognitively (eg, interpret their surroundings, avoid objects, elude opponents) while performing the physical activities that allow them to carry out the necessary active and reactive movements to prevent injuries during play. In addition to dual-tasking balance activities with sport-specific activities (eg, puck control, catching a ball), these exercises lend themselves to incorporate cognitive demands that include on-the-fly changes in responses (eg, switch hands used to catch a ball) or incorporating verbal, visual, and numeric memory activities to be performed concurrently. Figure 28-1 illustrates a sample progression of these activities.

An active approach to managing concussion may facilitate recovery and ease the patient's mind regarding losing fitness and being away from his or her sport. Recent evidence seems to indicate that light-to-moderate activity may aid in managing prolonged symptoms, vestibular rehabilitation may facilitate recovery in patients with vestibular symptoms, and dual tasking may engage the patient and aid cognitive recovery as well. It is important to note that any active rehabilitation should be symptom specific and supervised to ensure the patient tolerates the activities.

References

1. Giza CC, Hovda DA. The neurometabolic cascade of concussion. *J Athl Train*. 2001;36(3):228-235.
2. Leddy JJ, Kozlowski K, Donnelly JP, Pendergast DR, Epstein LH, Willer B. A preliminary study of subsymptom threshold exercise training for refractory post-concussion syndrome. *Clin J Sport Med*. 2010;20(1):21-27.
3. Alsalaheen BA, Mucha A, Morris LO, et al. Vestibular rehabilitation for dizziness and balance disorders after concussion. *J Neurol Phys Ther*. 2010;34(2):87-93.
4. Alsalaheen BA, Whitney SL, Mucha A, Morris LO, Furman JM, Sparto PJ. Exercise prescription patterns in patients treated with vestibular rehabilitation after concussion. *Physiother Res Int*. 2013;18(2):100-108.
5. Cicerone KD, Dahlberg C, Kalmar K, et al. Evidence-based cognitive rehabilitation: Recommendations for clinical practice. *Arch Phys Med Rehabil*. 2000;81(12):1596-1615.

WHICH PATIENT SELF-REPORT MEASURES ARE BEST FOR ASSESSING THE IMPACT OF CONCUSSION ON A PATIENT'S QUALITY OF LIFE?

Michelle L. Weber, MS, AT, ATC and
Tamara C. Valovich McLeod, PhD, ATC, FNATA

Self-reported outcomes measures are becoming increasingly popular in the assessment of how an illness or injury can impact a patient's perception of his or her health status, also known as health-related quality of life (HRQOL). These instruments allow insight into a broader spectrum of contemporary disablement models, such as the International Classification of Functioning. These measures allow patients to describe the impact of their injury on other aspects of their life, beyond the physical domain, including social, psychological, spiritual, economic, and work or school functioning. Typical concussion assessments have focused on impairments in cognition and balance; however, assessing how the injury is affecting other areas of their life is arguably just as important, if not more. The use of patient-reported outcome measures that evaluate the patient's perception of health outcomes can be important in understanding this perspective and helpful to the clinician in determining the best management practices for an individual patient.

Valovich McLeod TC, ed. *Quick Questions in Sport-Related Concussion: Expert Advice in Sports Medicine* (pp 145-151).
© 2015 Taylor & Francis Group.

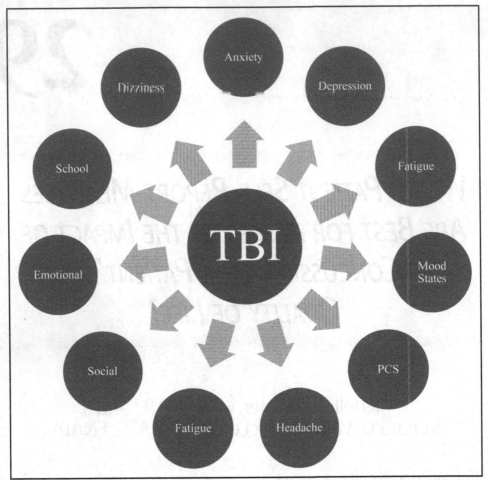

Figure 29-1. Areas of function and well-being that may be affected following concussion.

Concussions often result in vestibular dysfunction, postural control deficits, increased self-report symptoms, mental status deficits, and neurocognitive deficits. Currently, clinicians do a good job in following best practices to evaluate and manage those common areas affected by concussion. However, concussion can also result in myriad other issues that may not be captured by the traditional adjunct assessments (Figure 29-1) and warrant the inclusion of patient self-report outcome measures. Unlike patient self-report outcome measures for shoulder or knee injuries, where clinicians have 30 to 50 different instruments specific to that body part from which to choose, there is not one specific measure that has been developed for sport-related concussion. However, the many domains known to be affected by concussion can be assessed through generic or condition- or symptom-specific outcomes instruments, as well as self-report symptom inventories.[1,2] Some studies have begun to explore this area and have demonstrated associations between concussion and mood disturbances,[3] depression,[4,5] and global HRQOL[6] (see Figure 29-1).

Generic outcome measures can be used across illness and injuries and examine the overall HRQOL of the patient. Many have various subscales that can also be used to isolate specific aspects of HRQOL, such as social interactions or physical functioning. These measures include the Medical Outcomes Short Form (SF-36), a shorter version of the SF-36 called the SF-12, the Pediatric Quality of Life Inventory (PedsQL) generic scale, and the Patient Report Outcomes Measurement Information System (PROMIS) adult and pediatric profile instruments.

Disease-specific measures include the Quality of Life After Brain Injury (QOLIBRI) and Neuro-QOL. The QOLIBRI assesses satisfaction (cognition, self, daily life and autonomy, social relationships) as well as emotional and physical problems.[2] The Neuro-QOL is a group of self-report outcomes that assess HRQOL of patients with neurological disorders. This set of measures includes both generic instruments that can be used across many neurologic conditions and instruments for specific patient populations, such as stroke, epilepsy, and multiple sclerosis. The Neuro-QOL instruments examine mobility/ambulation, activities of daily living/upper extremity, depression, anxiety, positive psychological functioning, stigma, perceived and applied cognition, social role performance, social role satisfaction, fatigue, personality and behavioral change, and sleep disturbances, all of which may be applicable to concussed patients.[2]

Symptom-specific outcomes measures can be utilized when a clinician is aiming to evaluate the effect of one particular symptom on functioning in several disablement domains (Table 29-1). For example, a clinician who suspects a student-athlete is having trouble with depression during a prolonged recovery can choose the Beck Depression Inventory to gain an in-depth understanding of the patient perspective related to depression. Clinicians should determine which, if any, symptoms are most problematic for a patient following concussion and choose the symptom-specific patient-report outcome instrument accordingly.

The inclusion of patient-report outcomes for traumatic brain injury (TBI) practice and research is recommended by several organizations, including the Interagency TBI Outcomes Workgroup.[2] Several patient-report outcomes and HRQOL instruments are included as basic or supplemental common data elements that should be captured to obtain uniform information across all severity of TBIs, including concussion.

The recommended patient-report and HRQOL instruments are listed in Table 29-2. These instruments should accompany other tools being used, such as neurocognitive and balance assessments.

By adding patient-report outcome measures to the concussion assessment, clinicians may be able to identify possible issues that may hinder the patient's recovery

Table 29-1

Symptom-Specific Outcome Measures

Scale	Symptom Domains	Instrument Description
Beck Depression Inventory	Evaluates the intensity of depressive symptoms	21-item instrument scored on a 4-point Likert scale. Scores range from 0 to 63, with higher scores indicating increased severity of depression.
Dizziness Handicap Inventory	Evaluates the functional, emotional, and physical aspects of dizziness and unsteadiness	25-item instrument scored on a 3-point Likert scale. Scores range from 0 to 100, with higher scores indicating a greater impact of dizziness.
Headache Impact Test	Impact of headache on pain, social function, role function, vitality, cognitive function, and psychological distress	6-item scale, with each item scored on a 5-point Likert scale. A higher score indicates greater impact of headache on HRQOL.
Migraine Disability Assessment	Evaluates disability in family, social, and leisure activities as a result of migraine and migraine symptoms	5-item scale that asks the number of days lost over a 3-month period due to migraine symptoms. Higher scores indicate a greater effect on HRQOL.
Pediatric Migraine Disability Assessment	Impact of recurrent headache and migraine on the areas of school, participation in organized activities, and peer interactions	6-item instrument where patients report the number of days during the past 3 months when migraine has impacted HRQOL. Higher scores indicate greater effect of migraine on HRQOL.
Multidimensional Fatigue Scale	Impact of general, sleep, and cognitive fatigue on quality of life	18-item instrument using a 5-point Likert scale. Lower scores indicate greater impact of fatigue on HRQOL.
Profile of Mood States	Evaluates emotion through rating of moods: tension, vigor, depression, anger, fatigue, confusion, self-esteem	Brief instrument uses 40 adjectives organized into the 7 subscales. Responses on a 5-point Likert scale.

Table 29-2

Recommendations for the Use of Common Outcome Measures for Traumatic Brain Injury

Outcome Measure	Outcome Domain	Relevant Patient Population	Description of Domain
Neuro-QOL (www.neuroqol.org/Pages/default.aspx)	Patient-reported outcomes	Adult and pediatric	1C-item banks with Likert responses addressing the domains of anxiety, depression, stigma, positive psychological functioning, mobility, activities of daily living, satisfaction with social activities and roles, social roles, applied and perceived cognitive functioning
Patient-Reported Outcomes Measurement Information System (PROMIS) (www.nihpromis.org/default.aspx)	Patient-reported outcomes	Adult and pediatric	12-item banks with Likert responses addressing the domains of anger, anxiety, depression, fatigue, pain, physical function, satisfaction with social activities and roles, sleep/wake disturbance, and global health
Pediatric Quality of Life Inventory (PedsQL) (www.pedsql.org)	Perceived generic and disease-specific HRQOL	Pediatric (ages 5 to 18 years)	23-item instrument to assess HRQOL in children, including physical, emotional, social, and school functioning domains
Quality of Life after Brain Injury (QOLIBRI) (http://www.qolibrinet.com/)	Perceived generic and disease-specific HRQOL	Adult	37-item disease-specific instrument to measure HRQOL after traumatic brain injury, including 4 satisfaction scales (cognition, self, daily life and autonomy, and relationships), 2 bothered scales (emotions and physical problems), and a total score

(continued)

Table 29-2 (continued)

Recommendations for the Use of Common Outcome Measures for Traumatic Brain Injury

Outcome Measure	Outcome Domain	Relevant Patient Population	Description of Domains
Satisfaction With Life Scale (SWLS)	Perceived generic and disease-specific HRQOL	Adult	5-item instrument answered on a 7-point Likert scale
Health and Behavior Inventory (HBI)	TBI-related symptoms	Pediatric (with parent proxy)	20-item scale that measures the frequency of common concussion symptoms on a 4-point Likert scale
Postconcussion Symptom Inventory (PCSI)	TBI-related symptoms	Pediatric (ages 5 to 18 years)	Measures the degree to which each symptom is a problem for the patient in the areas of physical, cognitive, emotional, and sleep-related symptoms Different forms for each age range: age 5 to 7 (13 items), 8 to 12 (25 items), and 13 to 18 years (26 items)
Rivermead Postconcussive Symptom Questionnaire (RPQ)	TBI-related symptoms	Adult	16-item scale that measures the presence and severity of the symptoms on a 5-point Likert scale
Neurobehavioral Symptom Inventory (NSI)	TBI-related symptoms	Adult	22-item scale measuring the severity of each symptom on a 5-point Likert scale over the prior 2 weeks and results in a total score and cluster scores for physical, cognitive, affective, and sensory

Adapted from Wilde EA, Whiteneck GG, Bogner J, et al. Recommendations for the use of common outcome measures in traumatic brain injury research. Arch Phys Med Rehabil. 2010;91(11):1650-1660.e1617.

and assist in referral decisions, including the psychosocial and emotional ramifications of the concussion. Until a sport concussion–specific outcomes instrument is developed, outcome measures should be chosen based on the patient's presentation of symptoms and the treatment goals. By utilizing patient-report outcomes, clinicians can be assured that they are taking an individualized approach to managing their concussed patients and practicing in a manner exemplifying patient-centered care.

References

1. Valovich McLeod TC, Register-Mihalik JK. Clinical outcomes assessment for the management of sport-related concussion. *J Sport Rehabil.* 2011;20(1):46-60.
2. Wilde EA, Whiteneck GG, Bogner J, et al. Recommendations for the use of common outcome measures in traumatic brain injury research. *Arch Phys Med Rehabil.* 2010;91(11):1650-1660.e1617.
3. Hutchison M, Mainwaring LM, Comper P, Richards DW, Bisschop SM. Differential emotional responses of varsity athletes to concussion and musculoskeletal injuries. *Clin J Sport Med.* 2009;19(1):13-19.
4. Covassin T, Elbin RJ III, Larson E, Kontos AP. Sex and age differences in depression and baseline sport-related concussion neurocognitive performance and symptoms. *Clin J Sport Med.* 2012;22(2):98-104.
5. Guskiewicz KM, Marshall SW, Bailes J, et al. Recurrent concussion and risk of depression in retired professional football players. *Med Sci Sports Exerc.* 2007;39(6):903-909.
6. Valovich McLeod TC, Bay RC, Snyder AR. Self-reported concussion history affects health-related quality of life in adolescent athletes. *Athl Train Sports Health.* 2010;2(5):219-226.

SECTION V

RETURN TO ACTIVITY

WHY CAN'T AN ATHLETE RETURN TO PLAY ON THE SAME DAY AS THE CONCUSSION?

Scott C. Livingston, PhD, PT, ATC, SCS

The recognition, assessment, and management of concussions in sports has changed significantly over the past few decades as more attention has been focused on these mild traumatic brain injuries (mTBIs) across all levels of athletic competition. Current practice guidelines for the management of sports-related concussions are in agreement that an athlete diagnosed with a concussion or suspected of having a concussion cannot return to play (RTP) on the same day of injury. Full clinical and cognitive recovery must occur before consideration of RTP.[1-4] Potential health risks of returning a concussed athlete to play prior to complete recovery include the possibility of short-term complications and persistent or long-term health problems. This chapter will review the short-term risks associated with premature RTP, focusing on the increased susceptibility to further injury, delayed onset of postconcussion symptoms, a prolonged recovery period, and the possibility of second-impact syndrome (SIS). The potential for long-term complications resulting from a single or multiple episodes of repeated brain injuries will also be addressed.

Valovich McLeod TC, ed. *Quick Questions in Sport-Related Concussion: Expert Advice in Sports Medicine* (pp 155-158). © 2015 Taylor & Francis Group.

Short-Term Risks

There are numerous short-term risks associated with returning an athlete with persistent symptoms to play, including SIS and an increased susceptibility to a recurrent or more severe concussion with prolonged duration of symptoms. SIS involves diffuse cerebral swelling and occurs when an athlete sustains a second head injury before the signs and symptoms of the first concussion have fully cleared.[4] The pathophysiology of SIS involves a loss of autoregulation of the brain's blood supply leading to vascular engorgement, increased intracranial pressure, brain herniation, and coma or death. There is debate as to whether SIS is related to a prior head injury or if it represents a separate pathophysiological process of brain edema.[1] Whether or not a discrete entity of SIS exists, the association with concussion is a primary reason why an athlete should not return to play before symptoms of a concussion have completely resolved.[3]

Returning an athlete to play with persistent symptoms may also predispose him or her to a subsequent concussion, worse clinical presentation following any additional injury, and the potential for a protracted recovery period. While the brain heals from an initial concussive force, the risk for another injury is significantly higher. There is an increased risk of subsequent concussive injury that occurs with less force, especially if the time interval between injuries is short. The lower threshold of reinjury occurs in the first few days or weeks following initial injury. The window of vulnerability after a concussion is theorized to be the result of impaired cellular energy metabolism. A second injury before the brain has recovered results in worsening cellular metabolic changes and more significant cognitive deficits. Concussive injuries decrease cognitive ability and reaction time,[5] which may diminish an athlete's ability to respond to the demands of the sport, increasing the risk of a second brain injury. To diminish the risk of recurrent injury, individuals supervising athletes should prohibit an athlete with a concussive injury from returning to play/practice (contact-risk activity) until the athlete is asymptomatic (off medication), and until a licensed health care provider has judged that the concussion is resolved.

Practicing or playing a sport while still experiencing concussion symptoms can prolong the time to complete recovery and return to sports. Unlike other injuries in athletics, there may be significant consequences to "playing through" a concussion. When not treated promptly and properly, repetitive brain injuries can cause long-term problems. A longer cognitive recovery period may be necessary for younger athletes compared with college-aged or professional athletes,[5] often 7 to 10 days or longer. According to the American Academy of Pediatrics, because of the longer cognitive recovery time period among young athletes (even if the youth athletes are asymptomatic), a more conservative approach to RTP should be used.

Another primary short-term risk of premature RTP is the possibility of a delayed onset of signs and symptoms or neurologic decline in the acutely concussed athlete.

Table 30-1

Immediate and Delayed Symptoms of Concussion

Early or Immediate Symptoms	Late or Delayed Symptoms
Headache	Persistent low-grade headache
Dizziness	Lightheadedness
Lack of awareness of surroundings	Poor attention and concentration
Nausea or vomiting	Memory dysfunction
Any period of altered consciousness or amnesia	Easy fatigability
	Irritability
Changes in orientation	Anxiety, depressed mood, or other behavioral changes
Deficits in balance or coordination	
Diplopia	Sleep disturbance
Decreased reaction time	Alcohol intolerance
	Decreased performance on higher cognitive tasks

Adapted from Hough DO. Mild brain injury in sports. Proceedings of the Mild Brain Injury in Sports Summit, Washington, DC, April 16-18, 1994. National Athletic Trainers' Association Research & Education Foundation; 1994:31-41; and Guskiewicz KM, Bruce SL, Cantu RC, et al. National Athletic Trainers' Association position statement: management of sport-related concussion. *J Athl Train*. 2004;39(3):280-297.

At both the high school and collegiate levels, athletes may experience delayed neuropsychological deficits postinjury that are not evident on the sidelines and are also more likely to experience a delayed onset of symptoms.[5] Therefore, it is critical that the sports medicine clinician be able to differentiate between early or immediate symptoms (ie, those that develop within minutes to hours after the injury) and late or delayed symptoms (ie, symptoms that develop days to weeks after head trauma) (Table 30-1). The potential for a delayed onset of postconcussive signs and symptoms makes it imperative for the clinician to perform serial examinations of the concussed athlete.

Long-Term Risks

The long-term risks of premature RTP following concussion are the development of postconcussion syndrome, chronic traumatic encephalopathy (CTE), and chronic neurocognitive impairment (CNI). *Postconcussion syndrome* refers to persistent postconcussion symptoms lasting 3 months or longer and may be an indicator of concussion severity. The evolution of a concussive injury to postconcussion syndrome is ill defined and poorly understood, although several risk factors for postconcussion syndrome have been identified: increasing age, female sex, and nonsports–related mechanism of injury.[3] There is increasing concern that head-impact exposure and recurrent concussions may contribute to long-term neurological sequelae, including CTE and CNI. CTE is a neurodegenerative disease associated with repetitive head trauma, characterized by accumulation of tau protein in specific areas of the brain, resulting in executive dysfunction, memory impairment, depression, and poor impulse control. Factors other than repetitive head-impact exposure, such as a genetic predisposition, may lead to development of CTE.[1] CNI can present in postconcussion syndrome or may occur years after the last head injury. Evidence suggests that there is an increased risk of CNI with increased exposures to concussive forces and subconcussive blows to the head. Large-scale epidemiologic studies are required to clearly understand the causes of CTE and CNI and to develop prevention strategies.

Conclusion

A concussion is an *ongoing process* initiated by a physical force applied to the brain, and this process can last from hours to weeks. Sport-related brain injuries, even mild, represent a dynamic physiologic disruption of brain function in which the pathological picture evolves over minutes to hours to days after trauma and is characterized by a cascade of physiologic, vascular, and biochemical events. Because concussions are an *evolving injury* in the acute phase with rapidly changing clinical signs and symptoms, it is not always possible to rule out a concussion at the time of injury. The common view that a concussion is an injury that occurs at the time of impact and that symptom resolution and recovery proceed down a fixed but unpredictable path is inaccurate. During the recovery period, the clinician must limit any physiologic stressors (such as physical exertion, mental exertion, and sleep deprivation) and ensure that complete physiologic and clinical recovery has occurred before returning the athlete to sport.

References

1. McCrory P, Meeuwisse W, Johnston K, et al. Consensus statement on concussion in sport: the 3rd International Conference on Concussion in Sport held in Zurich, November 2008. *J Athl Train*. 2009;44(4):434-448.
2. Guskiewicz KM, Bruce SL, Cantu RC, et al. National Athletic Trainers' Association position statement: management of sport-related concussion. *J Athl Train*. 2004;39(3):280-297.
3. Harmon KG, Drezner JA, Gammons M, et al. American Medical Society for Sports Medicine position statement: concussion in sport. *Br J Sports Med*. 2013;47:15-26.
4. Herring SA, Cantu RC, Guskiewicz KM, Putukian M, Kibler WB. Concussion (mild traumatic brain injury) and the team physician: a consensus statement—2011 update. *Med Sci Sport Exerc*. 2011;43(12):2412-2422.
5. McCrea M, Guskiewicz KM, Marshall SW, et al. Acute effects and recovery time following concussion in collegiate football players: the NCAA Concussion Study. *JAMA*. 2003;290(19):2556-2563.

DOES RECOVERY FOLLOWING CONCUSSION FOLLOW A TYPICAL TIME COURSE, AND DOES THIS REALLY CORRESPOND TO RESOLUTION OF SELF-REPORTED SYMPTOMS?

Steven P. Broglio, PhD, ATC

For the majority of concussed male athletes, changes in postconcussion measures (eg, symptoms, balance, and neurocognitive functioning) will return to preinjury/baseline levels within 2 weeks following injury.[1] However, some research has demonstrated that the resolution of concussion symptoms does not correspond with the resolution of other commonly implemented concussion measures, such as neurocognitive assessments or functional imaging. For example, a group of 21 concussed collegiate athletes were evaluated during the preseason, within 72 hours of injury, and again when they no longer reported any concussion-related symptoms. Each assessment point included a computer-based neurocognitive evaluation and a symptom evaluation. As expected, the initial postconcussion assessment showed declines in neurocognitive performance in 81% of the sample. Surprisingly, the evaluation that took place once the athletes reported that they were asymptomatic (8.14 days postinjury) indicated that 38% continued to have a neurocognitive impairment.[2] A similar investigation evaluated 192 collegiate and high school participants (78 concussed symptomatic athletes, 44 concussed asymptomatic athletes, and 70 nonconcussed

Valovich McLeod TC, ed. *Quick Questions in Sport-Related Concussion: Expert Advice in Sports Medicine* (pp 159-161). © 2015 Taylor & Francis Group.

control athletes) on a computer-based neurocognitive evaluation. Performance on the computer evaluation showed the worst performance by the symptomatic group, followed by the asymptomatic athletes, and then the controls.[3] Together, these two studies suggest that cognitive impairment may continue beyond the point of symptom resolution, necessitating the use of sensitive measures of brain function.

Additional research adopting more sophisticated assessment measures has yielded similar results. In a small investigation implementing functional magnetic resonance imaging (fMRI), eight football athletes received a preseason fMRI evaluation while completing clinical measures for sequencing, a simple math task, and the digit-span task. Four of the athletes sustained concussions during the season and were rescanned using the same fMRI protocol within 1 week of the injury. At the postinjury assessment point, the concussed athletes showed a return to normal functioning on the clinical measures but continued to demonstrate irregular activation patterns on the fMRI scans.[4] This finding would suggest that despite a normal clinical presentation, subtle changes in cognitive functioning continued. Another investigation of cerebral activation in concussed athletes implemented magnetic resonance spectroscopy (MRS) in a group of 40 concussed athletes evaluated at days 3, 15, 22, and 30 postinjury. Similar to the fMRI investigation, the athletes reported becoming asymptomatic between the day 3 and day 15 evaluations. The MRS scans, however, indicated an altered cerebral metabolism up to 30 days following injury.[5]

Most recently, and perhaps most disconcerting, asymptomatic status without a concussion diagnosis may not necessarily mean alterations to cerebral activity have not occurred. A cohort of high school athletes were administered a preseason computerized neurocognitive evaluation and fMRI scan and were monitored for head impacts throughout the season. Four athletes were diagnosed with a concussion and evaluated within 72 hours. As expected, these individuals demonstrated depressed neurocognitive test performance and altered fMRI compared with their baseline. The investigators also evaluated a subset of the participants who had not reported concussion symptoms to the medical staff, nor did they have any outwardly visible signs of concussion. While this subgroup had a normal neurocognitive evaluation, it was found they displayed altered fMRI evaluations in absence of a concussion.[6] This finding would suggest that even without a concussion diagnosis, alteration to cerebral functioning can take place when an athlete is exposed to repeated subconcussive head impacts (ie, head impacts not resulting in concussion).

When viewed collectively, these findings suggest that concussed athletes who have reached asymptomatic status may continue to demonstrate deficits on neurocognitive evaluations commonly used in clinical practice. The return to preinjury levels of functioning may not necessarily mean that cerebral functional has been fully restored. One investigation reported altered activation patterns in the absence of cognitive deficits 1 week postinjury,[5] while another found that cerebral metabolism may be altered up to 30 days postinjury, despite symptom resolution between days 3 and 15.[5] Perhaps most alarming is the possibility that impacts to the head that do not result in concussion-like symptoms may result in altered cerebral activation but no changes to clinical performance.[6] Because the use of advanced imaging techniques remains largely research based and has not reached the point of clinical utility, clinicians should continue to approach concussion management in a multifaceted manner with neurocognitive and postural control measures used to support symptom reports and the clinical exam, as this approach offers the highest injury sensitivity.

References

1. McCrea M, Guskiewicz KM, Marshall SW, et al. Acute effects and recovery time following concussion in collegiate football players: the NCAA Concussion Study. *JAMA*. 2003;290(19):2556-2563.
2. Broglio SP, Macciocchi SN, Ferrara MS. Neurocognitive performance of concussed athletes when symptom free. *J Athl Train*. 2007;42(4):504-508.
3. Fazio VC, Lovell MR, Pardini JE, Collins MW. The relation between post concussion symptoms and neurocognitive performance in concussed athletes. *NeuroRehabilitation*. 2007;22(3):207-216.
4. Jantzen KJ, Anderson B, Steinberg FL, Kelso JA. A prospective functional MR imaging study of mild traumatic brain injury in college football players. *AJNR Am J Neuroradiol*. 2004;25(5):738-745.
5. Vagnozzi R, Signoretti S, Cristofori L, et al. Assessment of metabolic brain damage and recovery following mild traumatic brain injury: a multicentre, proton magnetic resonance spectroscopic study in concussed patients. *Brain*. 2010;133(11):3232-3242.
6. Talavage TM, Nauman EA, Breedlove EL, et al. Functionally-detected cognitive impairment in high school football players without clinically-diagnosed concussion. *J Neurotrauma*. 2014;31(4):327-338.

HOW LONG SHOULD PATIENTS BE FREE OF SYMPTOMS PRIOR TO BEGINNING A GRADUAL RETURN TO ACTIVITY?

Laura Decoster, ATC

The body of literature on sport concussion has expanded rapidly over the past 20 years. We know more now than ever before. Unfortunately, there are still many unanswered questions. Questions specific to the return-to-play (RTP) process are lacking evidence-based answers. In the absence of scientific answers to those questions, experts have convened to develop consensus. Indeed, today there are several areas of strong consensus. For example, it is widely agreed that athletes should not return to sports on the day a concussion occurs.[1-3] There is also consensus that no athlete should return to sports if he or she is still experiencing concussion signs or symptoms.[1,2,4] Beyond those 2 areas of agreement, there is agreement that certain presentations may represent red flags that should perhaps result in more conservative management. But there is limited consensus to support specific responses. This is true in all areas of the RTP discussion.

The RTP decision is still more art than science. The International Sport Concussion Group has long espoused a 5-step graduated RTP protocol.[2] According to the recent Zurich statement, the resolution of signs and symptoms is the

Valovich McLeod TC, ed. *Quick Questions in Sport-Related Concussion: Expert Advice in Sports Medicine* (pp 163-165).

appropriate launch point for gradual RTP.[2] There is a general recommendation that calls for a minimum of 24 hours between steps. However, there is no mention of requiring a symptom-free interval prior to beginning the RTP protocol.

Various themes for managing RTP have been advocated despite a lack of evidence of their efficacy, including the following:

- Once asymptomatic, a concussed athlete should wait for as many days as it took for symptoms to resolve prior to beginning the RTP protocol.

- Pediatric concussion patients should wait 7 days after symptoms resolve before starting the RTP protocol.

- Athletes with a history of previous concussions should add 3 days to the RTP protocol.

These ideas represent considerations that should contribute to your decision-making process. Others include the athlete's sport and comorbidities like migraines and attention deficit hyperactivity disorder (see Question 26). The wise clinician considers each athlete's history along with careful assessment of concussion signs and symptoms before making RTP decisions. Trying to manage concussions with a rule to wait 7 days may result in an athlete being returned too soon or too late. Starting the RTP protocol several days or weeks after symptom resolution might be the appropriate decision for one athlete, whereas starting immediately upon symptom resolution might be just as appropriate for another.

Although it is best to err on the side of caution, remember that rest has risks too. Judging the risks and benefits of activity is also important in the RTP process. Athletes should be carefully monitored as they progress through recovery. Plans and goals should be altered to accommodate observed improvement or regression.

A basic truth about concussion is that concussion severity and recovery defy neat categorization. No 2 concussions, or athlete responses to those concussions, are alike. The lack of objective diagnostic tools in current clinical use may be a factor here. Several promising diagnostic studies are being tested. Perhaps an objective measurement of concussion and its resolution is on the horizon. Having an objective means of recognizing concussion resolution would certainly help determine safe RTP. In the meantime, be sure to make decisions based on the presentation of each individual concussion.

References

1. Harmon KG, Drezner JA, Gammons M, et al. American Medical Society for Sports Medicine position statement: concussion in sport. *Br J Sport Med*. 2013;47(1):15-26.
2. McCrory P, Meeuwisse W, Aubry M, et al. Consensus statement on concussion in sport: the 4th International Conference on Concussion in Sport held in Zurich, November 2012. *J Sci Med Sport*. 2013;16(3):178-189.

3. Casa DJ, Almquist J, Anderson SA, et al. The inter-association task force for preventing sudden death in secondary school athletics programs: best-practices recommendations. *J Athl Train.* 2013;48(4):546-553.
4. American Academy of Neurology. AAN position statement on sports concussion. https://www.aan.com/PressRoom/Home/GetDigitalAsset/7952. Published October 2010. Accessed October 22, 2014.

WHAT IS THE ROLE OF THE GRADED EXERTION PROTOCOLS FOR MAKING RETURN-TO-PLAY DECISIONS?

Tracey Covassin, PhD, ATC and Jessica Wallace, MA, ATC, AT

When returning an athlete to participation, researchers and clinicians agree that a concussed athlete should never return to play on the same day as his or her concussion. Return to participation should be individualized and incorporate a multifaceted approach that includes athletes being symptom free, having a normal clinical neurological examination, and back to baseline measures on balance and neurocognitive measures. If brain imaging was performed, it should also be normal.

Over the past decade, our practice has changed for the concussed athlete. Previously, once an athlete was asymptomatic, we would return the athlete back to the playing field. More recent consensus statements now advocate for a stepwise return-to-play (RTP) criteria.[1] One of the main reasons we use stepwise RTP criteria is to make sure that athletes have completely healed so they are not at risk for second-impact syndrome (SIS), which can lead to permanent or catastrophic consequences. Moreover, RTP protocols are due to recognizing the need for the concussed athlete to engage in progressive physical and cognitive exertion with more activity day by day to see if symptoms emerge. Thus, some concussed athletes

Valovich McLeod TC, ed. *Quick Questions in Sport-Related Concussion: Expert Advice in Sports Medicine* (pp 167-169).
© 2015 Taylor & Francis Group.

Step	Rehabilitation Stage	Functional Exercise at Each Stage of Rehabilitation
	Table 33-1	
	Stepwise Return-to-Play Guidelines	
1	No activity	Complete cognitive and physical rest
2	Light aerobic exercise	Walking or stationary biking, intensity < 70% max heart rate, no weight training
3	Sport-specific activity	Shooting in basketball, running in soccer; no head impact activities
4	Noncontact training drills	Progress to more complex training drills (eg, passing drills in football); may commence weight training
5	Full-contact practice	Following medical clearance, participate in full-contact drills
6	Return to play	Normal game play

Adapted from McCrory P, Meeuwisse W, Aubry M, et al. Consensus statement on concussion in sport: the 4th International Conference on Concussion in Sport held in Zurich, November 2012. *Br J Sports Med.* 2013;47(5):250-258.

can be asymptomatic at rest, but once they start to exert and increase their heart rate and blood pressure, their symptoms will return. Therefore, we want to make sure we do not miss the athlete whose symptoms return due to exertion.

In 2000, the Canadian Academy of Sports Medicine Concussion Committee[2] was the original committee to develop a stepwise progression to return to participation. This stepwise RTP has been adopted by several consensus groups, including the International Concussion in Sport Group.[1] These stages are based on the possibility of symptoms returning from progressive physical and sport-specific exertion, which is why the concussed athlete should be medically supervised throughout the stepwise process. The recommended stepwise RTP process is outlined in Table 33-1. It is recommended that concussed athletes continue to proceed to the next level if they remain asymptomatic at the current stage. If concussion symptoms reappear, the athlete should revert to the previous asymptomatic stage and resume the progression after at least 24 hours of being asymptomatic. This progression can take anywhere from days to weeks or months, depending on the individual responses and modifying circumstances of each concussed athlete. It is also important to consider previous concussion history and duration of current symptoms when considering length of each stage. For example, an athlete who has 2 previous concussions may spend 3 to 4 days on each stage instead of the typical 24 hours between each stage.

When athletes are participating in a graded exertional protocol, the clinician should determine a symptom report not only during physical activity but also later in the day after exertion and the following morning. Therefore, when the concussed athlete returns 24 hours later, the clinician must make sure he or she was completely symptom free for the past 24 hours before proceeding to the next stage. Furthermore, graded exertional protocols must be individualized for each concussed athlete.

Although several consensus statements advocate for this stepwise RTP,[1,3] none of these graded exertional protocols has been validated with a double-blind prospective study. Moreover, researchers suggest that athletes who exhibit prolonged symptoms may start a graded exertional protocol at a lower level as long as symptoms are not exacerbated.[4] Thus, additional research is warranted to determine if a graded exertional protocol is supported by not only clinical practice but also by evidence-based practice.

References

1. McCrory P, Meeuwisse W, Aubry M, et al. Consensus statement on concussion in sport: the 4th International Conference on Concussion in Sport held in Zurich, November 2012. *Br J Sports Med.* 2013;47(5):250-258.
2. Canadian Academy of Sport Medicine Concussion Committee. Guidelines for assessment and management of sport-related concussion. *Clin J Sport Med.* 2000;10:209-211.
3. Harmon K, Drezner J, Gammons M, et al. American Medical Society for Sports Medicine position statement: concussion in sport. *Br J Sports Med.* 2013;47(1):15-26.
4. Makdissi M, Cantu R, Johnston K, McCrory P, Meeuwisse W. The difficult concussion patient: what is the best approach to investigation and management of persistent (> 10 days) post-concussive symptoms? *Br J Sports Med.* 2013;47:308-313.

How Should Return to Play Be Managed in Athletes With Comorbid Factors, Such as Attention Deficit Hyperactivity Disorder or Prior History of Concussion?

Christopher G. Vaughan, PsyD and Valerie Needham, MS

The decision whether or not to return an athlete to sports competition after concussion, referred to as return to play (RTP), is fundamentally about an assessment of risk. It is imperative to differentiate RTP from returning to exercise (or other "play-like" activities), whereby the former is associated with heightened risk for concussion, while the latter is associated with relatively minimal risk of additional injury. The RTP concept discussed herein is about a return to sports competition with known injury risk, not the return to moderate amounts of exercise sometimes recommended as therapeutic during the recovery process.

It is commonly recommended that RTP only occur after concussion symptoms resolve, and often after neuropsychological testing and balance assessment indicates no other postinjury effects. The consensus-based recommendation for youth athletes is that RTP should include a 5- to 7-day symptom-free period that includes a graduated progression of increasing levels of exercise.[1] Only after successful completion of this monitored RTP exercise protocol with no return of symptoms may an athlete be cleared for full participation (Figure 34-1).

Valovich McLeod TC, ed. *Quick Questions in Sport-Related Concussion: Expert Advice in Sports Medicine* (pp 171-175). © 2015 Taylor & Francis Group.

Return to Sports Guidelines
Following a Concussion - General

Athlete Name:_____   Completed By:_____

Following a concussion, to ensure the athlete has fully recovered, a medically supervised 5 STEP Gradual Return to Play program must be successfully completed (symptom-free) before final clearance to return

Instructions: The Gradual Return to Play (RTP) program is initiated only when the athlete has had no symptoms at rest for at least one to two days. Below are the 5 progressive steps that the athlete must complete when cleared for gradual return to play. Start with Step 1. Wait at least 24 hours (or longer) between each Step. Ask the athlete if any symptoms appeared over the past 24 hours. In the **RTP Status Box,** circle response, record date, and initials. If no symptoms are reported over the 24 hours, go to the next Step. If any symptoms return at any time during this program, stop working out. Rest until symptom-free for 24 hours. Then return to the previous level with no symptoms, and repeat that Step. If symptoms return or get worse, seek medical attention. All 5 Steps must be successfully completed (symptom-free), and FINAL WRITTEN MEDICAL CLEARANCE must be obtained before return to full competition.

RTP Status

Step 1: Light General Conditioning Exercises:
- **NO CONTACT**
- Begin with a sport specific warm up.
- Do a (15-20 minute) workout which can include: stationary bicycle, fast paced walking or light jog, rowing or freestyle swimming.

Step 1 Date:_____
Symptoms   No Symptoms
(Circle one)
Initials:_____

Step 2: General Conditioning and Sport Specific Skill Work; Individually:
- **NO CONTACT**
- Continue with the sport specific warm-up.
- Slowly increase intensity and duration of workout (20-30 minutes).
- Begin skill work within the workout.
- Begin sport specific skill work within the workout, but no spins, dives, or jumps.

Step 2 Date:_____
Symptoms   No Symptoms
(Circle one)
Initials:_____

STEP 3: General conditioning, skill work; individually and with a team-mate:
- **NO CONTACT**
- Continue with general conditioning (up to 60 minutes). Increase intensity and duration. Begin interval training.
- Continue with individual skill work.
- May begin skill work with a partner.
- May start beginner level spins, dives and jumps.

Step 3 Date:_____
Symptoms   No Symptoms
(Circle one)
Initials:_____

STEP 4: General conditioning, skill work and team drills:
- **NO CONTACT** Do not play live scrimmages.
- Resume regular conditioning and duration of practice.
- Increase interval training and skill work as required.
- Gradually increase skill level of spins, dives and jumps.
- Review team plays with no contact.

Step 4 Date:_____
Symptoms   No Symptoms
(Circle one)
Initials:_____

Step 5: Full Team Practice with Body Contact:
- Join team in a full practice with controlled body contact.
- If a full practice is completed with no symptoms, get Final Medical Clearance form signed. Give to the coach. You are ready to return to competition.

Step 5 Date:_____
Symptoms   No Symptoms
(Circle one)
Initials:_____

Final Medical Clearance Instructions: For final medical clearance, send this completed form to your medical provider at the successful completion of the 5-step program.
Provider: Email:
Phone: Fax:

Figure 34-1. Return-to-play exercise protocol. (Adapted from Gerard Gioia and Christopher Vaughan, SCORE Program at Children's National Health System.)

In the situation of an athlete with comorbid risk factors, such as attention deficit/hyperactivity disorder (ADHD) or other developmental conditions, migraine headaches, or a psychiatric condition, or with a history of multiple previous concussions, the treating clinician may choose a more conservative approach in managing RTP. A conservative approach to RTP often occurs when there is less confidence in the clinical assessment (including symptom status) or when it is believed that an individual may be at greater risk for reinjury or for sustaining a future brain injury that could lead to persisting problems. Being conservative typically implies an extended length of time for the RTP, possibly over a period of several weeks or longer, or engaging in mild-to-moderate exercise for an extended period of time before starting sport-specific activities and before returning to higher-risk competition.

Comorbid developmental (eg, attention or learning disorders), medical (eg, personal or family history of headaches), or psychiatric (eg, depression, anxiety, or sleep disorders) conditions may complicate the determination of a complete recovery in that symptoms seen in concussion may also be present prior to the injury. This presents a challenge to the clinician to determine which symptoms have deviated from normal, and whether these changes are due to the biological injury of the concussion or to situational factors secondary to the injury experience. A careful examination of the frequency, type, and severity of symptoms before the injury and gathering information on the likely course of these symptoms due to the situational events following a concussion (eg, increased headaches due to a disrupted sleep schedule, poor concentration and academic performance as a result of the stress of being behind on assignments) are required.

Concurrent developmental, medical, or psychiatric issues may also affect recovery and ultimately the timing for RTP, in that an underlying deviation of typical biology may predispose someone to a concussion, or the recovery process itself may become more difficult due to the condition. For example, a child with ADHD may engage in more risk-taking behaviors than children without ADHD, leading to an increased risk for a concussion. A student with a language-based learning disability may have to spend additional cognitive effort on learning, a process that in and of itself may ultimately prolong the injury. Lastly, individuals who are already vulnerable with personal or genetic risk factors for certain psychological or physical conditions may potentially encounter worse outcomes following single or multiple concussions. Due to these inherent vulnerabilities, clinicians may choose more conservative management for RTP for those individuals known to be at higher risk for certain conditions. It is important to emphasize that while avoiding concussion may seem prudent in the presence of comorbidities, individuals also achieve benefit from sports and exercise, and so careful consideration must also be given to negative consequences of restricting sports participation, not just to the consequences of concussion. This may be particularly true for younger athletes with a comorbidity, where participation in exercise may help to improve their academic performance and better manage their health and typical symptoms.

There is little evidence-based guidance for clinicians in managing RTP for individuals with multiple previous concussions. However, knowing that the most consistently reported risk for future concussions is a history of a previous concussion,[2] it is believed that individuals with multiple previous concussions are at greater risk for future concussions and therefore should be returned to play more cautiously.

The most frequent occurrence of successive concussions occurs shortly after the initial injury, often within the first 10 days,[2] Animal research on concussion has provided evidence that this window of biological vulnerability occurs more specifically during a period of decreased glucose metabolism following concussion.[3] However, beyond this initial period of physiologic vulnerability, there may be 2 different reasons for an increased rate of reccurrence of concussion. The first is that there remains a continued biologically based susceptibility, not readily identified in a typical clinical evaluation. This may be the result of a process of cumulative effect that is not yet understood or because a more severe neuropathophysiological injury occurred than is typically conceptualized. Indeed, newer and more sophisticated neuroimaging techniques may reveal certain pathophysiologic changes in some individuals with concussion but not in others.[4] The potential of this differentiated pathological process in some individuals with concussion challenges the assumption that all children with previous concussion are at greater future risk for concussion—at least based on biological risk. A second reason for a higher occurrence of additional concussion in some individuals may not be biological, but rather behavioral or situational. For example, the rate of exposure of force to the head may be greater for one individual than for another due to various factors (eg, position played, number of games/practices or sports, style of play, equipment). Individual body structure may yield different biomechanics as a result of being hit in the head and also should be considered as a potential cause for increased susceptibility to multiple concussions for only some individuals.

The health care provider should consider the management of RTP differently based on the indication of increased biologically based risk vs behaviorally based risk. A conservative approach to RTP, if returning at all, seems warranted for those with suspected persisting biological vulnerability. Changes to sport, style of play, or other situational factors may be effective for reducing risk for someone whose injury history is suggestive of behavioral risk, and complete retirement from a sport may not be necessary. An evaluation to assess for heightened concern for biological risk may include increasing length of recovery over successive injuries, sustained change in one's ability to complete educational or vocational tasks after presumed recovery from concussion, increased susceptibility to concussion from lower biomechanical force, or other significant disruptions in life following the prior concussion(s). Behavioral risk may become apparent during a careful clinical examination and based on history and timing of previous injuries, description of style of play or type of sport, or other described situational factors.

Conclusion

Management of RTP requires a good clinical assessment of the course of concussion recovery, as well as an understanding of relevant comorbidities and concussion history. A conservative RTP process should be considered in the context of known or unknown risk, as well as the benefit of participation in sport. A careful clinical examination with attention to key risk factors, along with a balanced understanding of the benefits of participation, will allow a clinician to make an appropriately informed and individually based decision on the management of RTP.

References

1. McCroy P, Meeuwisse WH, Aubry M, et al. Consensus statement on concussion in sport: the 4th International Conference on Concussion in Sport held in Zurich, November 2012. *Br J Sports Med*. 2012;47(5):250-258.
2. Giza CC, Kutcher JS, Ashwal S, et al. Summary of evidence-based guideline update: evaluation and management of concussion in sports: report of the guideline development subcommittee of the American Academy of Neurology. *Neurology*. 2013;80(24):2250-2257.
3. Prins ML, Alexander D, Giza CC, Hovda DA. Repeated mild traumatic brain injury: mechanisms of cerebral vulnerability. *J Neurotrauma*. 2013;30(1):30-38.
4. Bigler ED. Neuroimaging biomarkers in mild traumatic brain injury (mTBI). *Neuropsychol Rev*. 2013;30(8):657-670.

HOW DO HEAD IMPACT INDICATORS WORK, AND IS THERE VALUE IN RECOMMENDING THAT PATIENTS PURCHASE THEM?

Jason P. Mihalik, PhD, CAT(C), ATC and Robert C. Lynall, MS, ATC

Mild traumatic brain injury (mTBI) research has provided clinicians with useful information as it pertains to individual pieces of the proverbial concussion puzzle including, but not limited to, symptomatology, postural stability, and cognitive function. While these studies have provided us with important information and have changed the way many medical professionals manage brain injuries, a number of contemporary studies have investigated impact biomechanics and have sought to shed light on proposed injury thresholds for mTBI. A discussion of head impact indicators would be incomplete without a brief review of the biomechanical studies exploring these injury thresholds because they establish the fundamental core for developing these indicator technologies.

Does an Injury Threshold Exist?

The exploration of mTBI linear acceleration thresholds emerged in the early 1980s.[1] Linear acceleration of the brain may be defined as movement in a straight

Valovich McLeod TC, ed. *Quick Questions in Sport-Related Concussion: Expert Advice in Sports Medicine* (pp 177-181). © 2015 Taylor & Francis Group.

line through the brain's center of mass and is typically represented in the literature as a "g force," expressed relative to gravitational acceleration. For example, standing on the earth at sea level imposes 1 g acceleration on a person. The g forces experienced by those on rollercoasters can range from 3.5 to 6.3 g (or acceleration equal to 3.5 to 6.3 times the acceleration due to gravity; 9.81 m/s²). These g forces are considerably lower than those employed by head impact indicators. It should be noted that high g forces related to head impact biomechanics are sustained over very short time durations (eg, 8 to 12 milliseconds) and are not sustained over longer periods of time (ie, seconds) experienced during rollercoasters or aerobatic flying. In context, the linear acceleration of a crash-test dummy head in a 35-mph frontal car collision is approximately 70 g.

During the 1980s, Hugenholtz and Richard[2] proposed an mTBI linear acceleration injury threshold of 80 to 90 g. In more contemporary studies, researchers have continued to explore the notion of an mTBI injury threshold. Laboratory reconstruction of concussive events captured from National Football League (NFL) game footage suggested that mTBI in helmeted sports are likely to occur between 70 and 75 g.[3] Several NFL head injuries were subsequently analyzed using the Wayne State University Brain Injury Model—a computer-simulated finite element model—reporting that resultant linear accelerations of the head center of gravity of 106 g were associated with an 80% probability of mTBI.[4]

As theoretical mTBI thresholds continue to emerge in the research literature, clinical research efforts in this area are indicating that such a simplistic threshold value is not realistic.[5] For example, previously published data[6] studying head impact biomechanics in college football players identified only 7 of 1858 head impacts exceeding an 80-g threshold (less than 0.38%) resulted in an mTBI diagnosis. While real-time accelerometer data collection is a novel approach to better understand mTBI biomechanics, a full comprehension of the biomechanical inputs of mTBI remains unknown. Unfortunately, these data are widely ignored by many manufacturers developing head impact indicator products.

How Do Head Impact Indicators Work?

We should begin this section by operationalizing the definition of *work*. We will discuss work in the context of how the equipment operates. To date, there have been no studies published on validity (measures accurately what it is purported to measure) or reliability (measures an outcome consistently). There are many instruments currently on the market. A nonexhaustive list is provided in Table 35-1. In short, there are 2 primary types: (1) pure indicators and (2) measurement/monitoring systems.

Table 35-1
Head Impact Indicators

Manufacturer	Brand Name	Attachment	Threshold
Battle Sports Science, LLC	Impact Indicator 2.0	Chinstrap	240 HIC
gForce Tracker, Inc	gForce Tracker*	Helmet	Programmable threshold
Heads-Up Stabilizer	First Alert Concussion Sensor	Helmet	Unspecified g level
Impakt Protective, Inc	Shockbox	Helmet	Yellow light at 50 g, orange light at 90 g
Reebok International, Ltd and MC10, Inc	Checklight	Skullcap	Red and yellow LED lights, unknown threshold
Riddell	Head Impact Telemetry System*	Helmet	Programmable threshold
Riddell	InSite Impact Response System	Helmet	3 factors: (1) position, (2) skill level, (3) single impact in top 1% (HITsp) or multiple impacts in 7-day period in top 5%
Triax Technologies LLC	Smart Impact Monitor*	Headband or skullcap	Programmable threshold
X2 Biosystems	xPatch*	Head	Programmable threshold

Abbreviation: HIC, Head Injury Criterion.
*Capable of functioning as both an indicator and monitoring device.

Indicators are built with sensors capable of measuring the force (or velocity or acceleration) following a head impact and compare this value against a preprogrammed threshold. If an impact does not exceed the preprogrammed threshold, the impact is ignored and no indication is triggered. Conversely, when an impact exceeds a preprogrammed threshold, the device triggers an alert. The alerts can take on different forms ranging from, but not limited to, a visual alert on the device itself (eg, a flashing light), an audible alert emanating from the device (eg, a beep or buzzing indicator), or an alert delivered to an external device (eg, tablet,

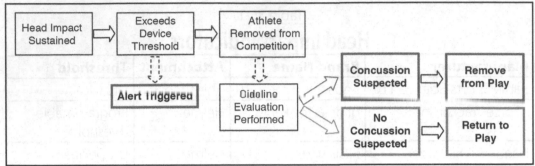

Figure 35-1. Recommended end-user action following an alert.

handheld device). Some indicators prompt the end user—a coach, parent, player, or sideline clinician—to perform an evaluation before he or she is able to reset the device and prime it for the next trigger-related head impact. Figure 35-1 displays the manufacturer-recommended action to be taken by the end user after an alert is triggered. Indicators are limited in their ability to provide meaningful data to clinical researchers. There are rarely any data collected on nonthreshold triggering events that can be studied. Because we know very little of the biomechanical inputs of mTBI, clinical researchers can continue to learn as much from impacts that do not cause injury as we can from those that result in an mTBI diagnosis. Additionally, many indicators have not been validated in independent laboratory testing. With no numerical outputs and lack of validation, it is difficult to ascertain the true magnitude of a trigger event.

Measuring or monitoring systems may provide some indication of head impact severity but are distinct from indicator systems in that they are capable of measuring, storing, and exporting vast clinical research data for future study. Such systems that have been widely used in clinical research include the Head Impact Telemetry (HIT) System and the devices manufactured by X2 Biosystems. Both have built-in notifications (eg, paging alerts), and they have collectively provided clinical researchers with valuable field data from over 2 million individual head impacts.

Patient Recommendations

In order for a clinical tool to be recommended, it must possess certain characteristics. It must be valid, reliable, sensitive (correctly identify a patient with a condition when the person actually has the condition), and specific (correctly identify a patient as not having a condition when the person actually does not have the condition). Additionally, a clinical tool must possess high positive predictive value. A head impact indicator would be deemed to possess a high positive predictive value—and thus clinical usefulness—if there was a high likelihood that an impact triggering an alert resulted in a diagnosed mTBI.

In our own work, we have studied the clinical usefulness of head impact indicators at various threshold levels.[7] For the sake of demonstration, assume that one device in particular employs a conservative injury threshold (approximately 100 g). Our head impact biomechanics data suggest that it would only possess 46% sensitivity, meaning the indicator would have only triggered an alert for 46% of all diagnosed concussions, thus missing 54% of all cases. Our same data would indicate an almost nonexistent positive predictive value of 0.4%. This means that of all impacts exceeding the preprogrammed 100-g threshold (n = 2828), only 0.4% (n = 11) would have resulted in a diagnosed mTBI; thus, a head impact indicator employing a 100-g threshold would yield a *99.6% false-positive rate*. Although the numbers may change slightly based on particular parameters employed by different head impact indicators, the overall story remains the same: they have not been validated, they have not been shown to be reliable, and their clinical usefulness (or lack thereof) does not justify the financial, human, and physical resources required to operate and maintain them. Additionally, one theme is beginning to emerge from the research: head injuries may be more likely influenced by a combination of the magnitude and frequency of head impacts and not by a single head impact. Until such time as the biomechanical inputs of head trauma are fully understood, head impact indicators should be employed with extreme caution.

References

1. Hodgson VR, Thomas LM, Khalil TB. The role of impact location in reversible cerebral concussion. *Proceedings of the 27th Stapp Car Crash Conference.* Warrendale, PA: Society of Automotive Engineers; 1983:225-240.
2. Hugenholtz H, Richard MT. Return to athletic competition following concussion. *Can Med Assoc J.* 1982;127(9):827-829.
3. Pellman EJ, Viano DC, Tucker AM, Casson IR, Waeckerle JF. Concussion in professional football: reconstruction of game impacts and injuries. *Neurosurgery.* 2003;53(4):799-812.
4. Zhang L, Yang KH, King AI. A proposed injury threshold for mild traumatic brain injury. *J Biomech Eng.* 2004;126(2):226-236.
5. Guskiewicz KM, Mihalik JP. Biomechanics of sport concussion: quest for the elusive injury threshold. *Exerc Sport Sci Rev.* 2011;39(1):4-11.
6. Mihalik JP, Bell DR, Marshall SW, Guskiewicz KM. Measurement of head impacts in collegiate football players: an investigation of positional and event-type differences. *Neurosurgery.* 2007;61(6):1229-1235.
7. Lynall RC, Mihalik JP, Guskiewicz KM, Marshall SW. The validity of head impact indicators to positive predict concussion. *J Athl Train.* 2013;48(3):S153.

SECTION VI

RETURN TO SCHOOL

WHAT IS COGNITIVE REST, AND CAN IT HELP RECOVERY FOLLOWING CONCUSSION?

Christopher G. Vaughan, PsyD and Valerie Needham, MS

Cognitive and physical rest has been considered the cornerstone of concussion treatment for the past decade.[1] The concept of cognitive rest is based on the premise that increased cognitive activities following concussion stress the dysfunctional neurometabolic system of the brain in a way that impedes recovery.[2] In theory, systematically reducing cognitive activities enables increased brain rest, thereby enabling the dysfunctional neurometabolic system to return to normal and to facilitate a faster recovery from concussion. Despite the consensus that cognitive rest should be recommended, there is only limited empirical support that cognitive activities prolong recovery or that cognitive rest would therefore shorten recovery.[3]

In a recent review of evidence examining the use of rest following concussion in sport,[4] only 3 studies meeting inclusion criteria were identified pertaining to cognitive rest. A single prospective treatment study of high school and college athletes showed improved cognition and symptoms following prescribed recommendations for cognitive and physical rest, regardless of time since injury.[5] However, the absence of a contrast group in this study leaves open the possibility that these improvements

Valovich McLeod TC, ed. *Quick Questions in Sport-Related Concussion: Expert Advice in Sports Medicine* (pp 185-188).
© 2015 Taylor & Francis Group.

were due to factors other than the recommendation of rest specifically or that rest may improve symptom report and cognitive function in any population, not just individuals with concussion. Two retrospective studies supported the use of rest as a benefit for symptoms following concussion, although these were also without well-controlled or equated contrast groups.[4]

The potential negative outcomes of cognitive rest following concussion also need to be considered, particularly if used for extended periods of time or to an extreme. Recommending restrictions to daily activities that involve the brain can theoretically be infinite, and potential consequences to such restrictions including depression, anxiety, social withdrawal, irritability, and acting-out behavior have been raised.[4] Physical symptoms such as headaches may actually increase as a result of reducing mental activities, as pain awareness can increase without activities to serve as an active distraction. Prescribing rest may therefore limit an opportunity to engage in coping activities that could serve as a beneficial distraction from unpleasant symptoms. Increased anxiety as a result of avoiding school or work is also a concern. When unpleasant symptoms are initially reduced by avoiding certain activities, attempts to return to those activities may initially lead to an increase in anxiety and ultimately in symptoms. Lastly, activities that are perceived to be restful may instead lead to significant increases in stress (eg, falling behind in school or work), and this stress response may counteract any potential physiological benefit of rest.

Cognitive rest as a treatment remains a poorly defined concept, making it difficult to study empirically. An activity viewed by some as mentally active (eg, watching television, reading) may be viewed by others as pleasurable and relaxing. Similarly, activities may have a relaxing effect for short periods of time but become tiring over extended periods of time. The benefit of cognitive rest may also have a limited temporal window. Physical rest, theoretically recommended for similar reasons, appears to have maximal benefit early after concussion, but not for prolonged periods of time. Indeed, one study showed that voluntary physical exercise, when implemented at a postacute period following concussion, actually improved cognitive outcomes in rodents.[6] In this animal model, brain-derived neurotrophic factor (BDNF), a protein that supports the health and growth of neurons in the brain, was increased following voluntary exercise and was associated with improved memory performance in rats. An analogous human study of appropriately timed cognitive exercise has not been examined to our knowledge, although the beneficial health mechanisms of physical exercise are likely to be different from the benefit of cognitive activity.

Fortunately, cognitive activities and cognitive rest exist on a continuum and are not diametrically opposed. Therefore, the use and prescription for cognitive rest can, and probably should, occur across a gradient.[2] Greater restriction from activities may be more appropriate earlier after an injury, with a progressive increase in activities as time from injury increases. One pragmatic justification for the

Cognitive Activity Monitoring (CAM) Log

Name_____   Parent/ Teacher:_____

DATE **TIME**							
LOCATION (circle one)	Home School	Home School	Home School	Home School	Home School	Home School	Home School
COGNITIVE ACTIVITY:							
DURATION:							
SYMPTOM (PRE/POST) HEADACHE FATIGUE CONCENTRATION PROBLEMS IRRITABILITY FOGGINESS LIGHT/ NOISE SENSITIVITY Other:_____	Rate 0-10 __/__ __/__ __/__ __/__ __/__ __/__ __/__	Rate 0-10 __/__ __/__ __/__ __/__ __/__ __/__ __/__	Rate 0-10 __/__ __/__ __/__ __/__ __/__ __/__ __/__	Rate 0-10 __/__ __/__ __/__ __/__ __/__ __/__ __/__	Rate 0-10 __/__ __/__ __/__ __/__ __/__ __/__ __/__	Rate 0-10 __/__ __/__ __/__ __/__ __/__ __/__ __/__	Rate 0-10 __/__ __/__ __/__ __/__ __/__ __/__ __/__
PRE-POST DIFFERENCE	———	———	———	———	———	———	———

G. Gioia, PhD 2012

CAM Log Instructions

1. Record the time and day of the activity monitoring.
2. Circle the location – home or school (or other)
3. Briefly describe the cognitive activity (e.g., math homework, pleasure reading, puzzle)
4. Indicate the length of time of the activity in minutes or hours
5. Before starting the activity, rate the 6 symptoms on a scale of 0 (not present) to 10 (highest symptom level). At the end of the session, rate the symptoms again from 0-10. If there is another key symptom, write it in and rate it before and after the activity.
6. Total the 6 pre-Activity ratings, and total the 6 post-Activity ratings. Calculate the difference.

Figure 36-1. Cognitive activity monitoring log. (Reprinted with permission from Gerard Gioia, PhD.)

recommendation for cognitive rest following concussion is that many symptoms increase after concussion as a result of sustained cognitive activities. Symptoms may become less distressing and unpleasant by avoiding activities that cause them, thereby improving an individual's quality of life during the time of recovery, regardless of whether the rest actually helps to physiologically promote the recovery.

Following the acute phase after injury, a controlled and graduated return to activities is often recommended. Determining cognitive or psychosocial triggers for symptoms on an individualized basis allows a treating provider to promote restful activities without implementing broad-based restrictions that may or may not have benefit. Utilizing a symptom-monitoring log (Figure 36-1) is encouraged to help identify which activities, and at what length of time, increase symptoms. A minimal increase (1 or 2 symptom points) may be tolerable, while a more significant increase may warrant modifications to the activity. This log can also serve to identify other activities that are well tolerated and can be encouraged. A significant restriction in activities should only be made after careful consideration is given to the importance of the activities (eg, school/work), the potential value of the activity as a coping mechanism (eg, maintaining a regular routine), and based on the individual's perception of the consequence or benefit of avoiding the particular cognitive activity. Furthermore, rest can be recommended in response to certain activities only when symptoms worsen, but it should be acknowledged that some increase in "symptoms" may be a typical experience and may not justify complete avoidance from a difficult activity.

Overall, it remains recommended that the goal of any provider recommending rest should be to return the individual to normal activities as early as possible following concussion.[3] Individual factors should be considered when recommending cognitive restrictions and rest using a practical but cautious approach until more concrete evidenced-based practice becomes available.

References

1. McCrory P, Meeuwisse WH, Aubry M, et al. Consensus statement on concussion in sport: the 4th International Conference on Concussion in Sport held in Zurich, November 2012. *Br J Sports Med.* 2012;47(5):250-258.
2. Valovich McLeod TC, Gioia GA. Cognitive rest: the often neglected aspect of concussion management. *Athlet Ther Today.* 2010;15(2):1-3.
3. Halstead ME, McAvoy K, Devore CD, et al. Returning to learning following concussion. *Pediatrics.* 2013;132(5):948-957.
4. Schneider KJ, Iverson GL, Emery CA, McCrory P, Herring SA, Meeuwisse WH. The effects of rest and treatment following sport-related concussion: a systematic review of the literature. *Br J Sports Med.* 2013;47(5):304-307.
5. Moser RS, Glatts C, Schatz P. Efficacy of immediate and delayed cognitive and physical rest for treatment of sports-related concussion. *J Pediatr.* 2012;161(5):922-926.
6. Griesbach GS, Hovda DA, Gomez-Pinnilla F. Exercise-induced improvement in cognitive performance after traumatic brain injury in rats is dependent on BDNF activation. *Brain Res.* 2009; 1288:105-115.

HOW CAN CONCUSSION NEGATIVELY AFFECT SCHOOL FUNCTIONING?

Danielle M.E. Ransom, PsyD and
Christopher G. Vaughan, PsyD

Developing new academic skills is a central component of child and adolescent development. School functioning predominantly refers to this academic learning but also entails navigating complex social situations and independently managing the academic demands themselves. Acknowledging that school functioning is a concept much broader than just academic skills, this chapter will predominantly focus on what is known and theorized to be the impact of concussion on school academics.

Concussion threatens a student's ability to learn and achieve academically in several ways. First, learning may be directly impeded by the symptoms themselves (eg, headaches, fatigue), including the cognitive effects of the brain injury (eg, impaired concentration, slowed processing speed). Second, the symptoms of concussion, and sometimes the recommended treatment, may require absence from school for a period of time. Limited access to instruction interferes with a student's ability to keep pace with new learning. Third, efforts to engage in challenging cognitive

Valovich McLeod TC, ed. *Quick Questions in Sport-Related Concussion: Expert Advice in Sports Medicine* (pp 189-194).
© 2015 Taylor & Francis Group.

activities soon after concussion may lead to worsened symptoms (sometimes called *cognitive exertion effects*). Receiving instruction during symptoms, and particularly when those symptoms increase with effort to overcome them, further exacerbates a cycle of learning problems and school absences. The mechanisms for these effects of concussion on school learning, along with relevant treatment recommendations and clinical issues, are discussed below.

Fundamental to school are the requirements that students gain new knowledge, develop and practice various academic skills, and complete work within a limited amount of time. Success in school therefore relies on a student's ability to divide attention among competing demands in the classroom, learn and recall course-specific content, and generate and apply problem-solving approaches to accomplish novel tasks—often across multiple subjects. These cognitive skills, including attention, learning and memory, processing speed, and executive functions (eg, flexibility, planning, and problem solving), have been shown to be impacted by concussion.[1] Indeed, disruption in any cognitive domain has the potential to impair learning and overall academic achievement. In an unpublished sample of children aged 5 to 18 years with concussion gathered through our specialty concussion clinic, a majority of students (66%) after concussion reported that headaches interfered with school learning. Concentration problems, difficulties with new learning or memory, and feeling too tired to engage in academic tasks were also reported.[2] Less commonly, the presence of other symptoms (eg, sleep disturbance, light/noise sensitivity, dizziness, visual problems) may also disrupt a student's participation in school activities.

School absences following concussion may also have a significant and negative impact on learning and academic functioning. Although initial absence may be necessary after the injury due to the severity of the symptoms, prolonged absence from school is not advised. As stated in a recent consensus opinion and review of pediatric concussion, it is recommended that youth return to typical activities (including school) as soon as possible after injury.[3] Students who miss periods of school following concussion face demands to keep pace with new learning and assignments while making up for missed academic work. This duel challenge of new learning plus completing missed work can be overwhelming for many students. In our experience, students faced with the burden of significant make-up work occurring at the same time as having heightened concussion symptoms often do not fare well unless school accommodations and supports are provided.

Conversely, to avoid the consequences of falling behind in schoolwork, symptomatic students often attempt to maintain their usual workload despite the presence of these symptoms. The cognitive demands of certain school-related activities may provoke concussion symptoms, which in turn further interferes with new learning and academics. This can be overwhelming for students, particularly those with high academic expectations, when they are not capable of functioning at full capacity. In the case of either a student failing to keep pace with a progressively increasing list of assignments or one who has maintained his or her workload but is performing at a level below typical expectations, emotional consequences such as depression or anxiety can occur.[4]

General guidance on "returning to learning" was recently published and highlighted the need to balance management of concussion symptoms with return to the academic environment.[3] However, these recommendations largely remain theoretical with little empirical support. Service delivery for students with a concussion remains one of the biggest challenges, as existing school-based support mechanisms (ie, 504 plan, Individualized Education Plan) may not fit this injury due to the need for monitoring and modifications to the support plan based on the evolving recovery. Individual differences further complicate making accommodations standardized, as the type and level of tolerable activity will vary from student to student after concussion. Characterizing the nature and extent of individual academic problems and symptom triggers is recommended to guide an individualized school-based support plan while maximizing a student's ability to participate in, and complete, learning requirements. Procedures guiding the gradual return to school are provided in Table 37-1 and may be implemented flexibly depending on students' symptoms and academic needs (eg, a student in the acute stage of recovery who is highly symptomatic may begin at step 0 or 1, while a student with minimal to moderate symptoms may begin at step 2, 3, or 4).

It is a multifaceted challenge to treat students recovering from concussion. Cognitive rest early after injury likely reduces symptom burden and possibly facilitates faster recovery (see Question 36) but often requires a temporary reduction in academic activities. During this time of rest, school absences and limitations placed on workload must not simultaneously leave students with an insurmountable workload or put them in significant distress at the prospect of real or perceived make-up work. A recommended therapeutic treatment approach relies on providing temporary school accommodations (Table 37-2) that strike a careful balance between participation in cognitive activities that do not significantly exacerbate symptoms and maintenance of the typical workload and assignment schedule as closely as possible.

Conclusion

Concussions can affect students by causing symptoms that impede new learning while also causing symptoms that interfere in classroom functioning. Mandatory school absence following concussion, or clinician-recommended treatment designed to minimize symptom exacerbation by avoiding school activities, may further remove students from the learning environment and compromise their

Table 37-1

Gradual Return to Academics

Stage	Description	Activity Level	Criteria to Move to Next Stage
0	No return, at home	Day 1: Maintain low-level cognitive and physical activity. No prolonged concentration. Cognitive readiness challenge: As symptoms improve, try reading or math challenge task for 10 to 30 minutes; assess for symptom increase.	(1) Student can sustain concentration for 30 minutes before significant symptom exacerbation, AND (2) Symptoms reduce or disappear with cognitive rest breaks* allowing return to activity
1	Return to school, partial day (1 to 3 hours)	Attend 1 to 3 classes, with interspersed rest breaks. Minimal expectations for productivity. No tests or homework.	Student symptom status improving, able to tolerate 4 to 5 hours of activity with 2 to 3 cognitive rest breaks built into school day
2	Full day, maximal supports (maximal supports required throughout day)	Attend most classes, with 2 to 3 rest breaks (20 to 30 minutes), no tests. Minimal homework (≤ 60 minutes). Minimal-moderate expectations for productivity.	Number and severity of symptoms improving, needs only 1 to 2 cognitive rest breaks built into school day
3	Return to full day, moderate supports (moderate supports provided in response to symptoms during day)	Attend all classes with 1 to 2 rest breaks (20 to 30 minutes); begin quizzes. Moderate homework (60 to 90 minutes). Moderate expectations for productivity. Design schedule for makeup work.	Continued symptom improvement, needs no more than one cognitive rest break per day

(continued)

Table 37-1 (continued)
Gradual Return to Academics

Stage	Description	Activity Level	Criteria to Move to Next Stage
4	Return to full day, minimal supports (monitoring final recovery)	Attend all classes with 0 to 1 rest break (20 to 30 minutes); begin modified tests (breaks, extra time). Homework (90 + minutes). Moderate-maximal expectations for productivity.	No active symptoms, no exertional effects across the full school day
5	Full return, no supports needed	Full class schedule, no rest breaks. Maximal expectations for productivity. Begin to address makeup work.	N/A

*Cognitive rest break: a period during which the student refrains from academic or other cognitively demanding activities, including schoolwork, reading, TV/games, and conversation. May involve a short nap or relaxation with eyes closed in a quiet setting.
Reproduced with permission from Gerard Gioia, MD.

Table 37-2
Accommodations for School-Related Postconcussion Effects

School-Related Problem	Potential Causes	Accommodation/ Management Strategy
Headaches interfering	Reduced tolerance for extended periods of concentration	Rest breaks alternating with gradually increasing periods of concentration
Problems with attention	Sleep disturbance, headache, decreased activation to engage in basic attention and working memory	Shorter assignments, break down tasks, decrease workload
Feeling too tired	Decreased arousal, shifted sleep schedule, cognitive exertion	Later school start time, shortened day
Increased time spent on homework	Problems accessing learned information when needed, fatigue	Rest breaks during academic activities (classes, homework, and exams)

(continued)

	Table 37-2 (continued)	
Accommodations for School-Related Postconcussion Effects		
School-Related Problem	**Potential Causes**	**Accommodation/ Management Strategy**
Difficulty understanding material	Problems keeping pace with work demand, difficulty processing verbal information effectively	Extended time on assignments and tests, slow down verbal information, comprehension checks
Difficulty studying	Diminished memory consolidation/retrieval	Smaller chunks to learn, recognition cues, no significant or standardized tests
Difficulty taking class notes	Problems holding new information in mind, comprehending new material, and dividing attention	Repetition, written instructions, teacher notes

Adapted from Sady MD, Vaughan CG, Gioia GA. School and the concussed youth: recommendations for concussion education and management. *Phys Med Rehabil Clin N Am.* 2011;22(4):701-719.

ability to manage the ongoing academic curriculum. Clinicians are faced with the challenge of balancing recommendations to minimize a student's symptom burden with the student's need to manage ongoing academic demands. A program that promotes a gradual return to school coupled with academic supports to reduce symptom burden may provide the ideal balance of these 2 objectives. Empirically derived guidelines are still needed to address students' postinjury academic needs.

References

1. Belanger HG, Vanderploeg RD. The neuropsychological impact of sports-related concussion: a meta-analysis. *J Int Neuropsychol Soc.* 2005;11(4):345-357.
2. Ransom D, Vaughan CG, Pratson L, et al. Effects of concussion on academic functioning and performance: a developmental perspective. Poster presented at: Inaugural Sports Neuropsychology Society Meeting and Symposium; May 3-4, 2013; Minneapolis, MN.
3. Halstead ME, McAvoy K, Devore CD, et al. Returning to learning following concussion. *Pediatrics.* 2013;132(5):948-957.
4. Iverson GL. Outcome from mild traumatic brain injury. *Curr Opin Psychiatry.* 2005;18(3):301-317.

WHAT SCHOOL POLICIES/PROCEDURES APPLY TO CONCUSSED STUDENT-ATHLETES WHO ARE ATTEMPTING TO RETURN TO THE CLASSROOM?

John T. Parsons, PhD, ATC and Richelle M. Williams, MS, ATC

To understand the policies and procedures that exist to assist a concussed student in returning to the classroom, one must understand the comprehensive impact of the concussion on the student's ability to fulfill his or her role in the classroom. Students with sport-related concussion (SRC) struggle with myriad physical, behavioral, and social issues that can significantly impact their ability to return to the classroom.[1] For example, physical issues may include headache, light sensitivity, and difficulty concentrating. Behavioral issues may include agitation, depression, and inappropriate behaviors.[2] Collectively, these issues may interfere with the person's ability to function as a student—to maintain the expected social role of "student." From that perspective, it can be argued that the concussed student is dealing with a disability, at least for as long as the signs and symptoms of the concussion remain.

Disability has been defined as "limitations in the socially defined roles and activities within a sociocultural and physical environment."[3] In this case, the

Valovich McLeod TC, ed. *Quick Questions in Sport-Related Concussion: Expert Advice in Sports Medicine* (pp 195-198).

sociocultural and physical environment is the classroom, which is a central location in the life of a school-aged student. Within the context of the student-athlete, a return to the classroom is also an important milestone in the management of a SRC because return-to-play progressions should not begin until the student is able to return to the classroom successfully.[2]

In the United States, the educational needs of disabled students have been managed through a variety of policy tools that can be collectively referred to as "educational accommodations." Accommodations can take varying forms depending on the nature of the disability and the classroom challenges that the disability presents to the student. They can be classified as both formal and informal and can be implemented either temporarily or permanently. Temporary education accommodations fall into 2 categories: (1) academic adjustments and (2) academic accommodations.[4] The third category, academic modification, is the permanent form of assistance, resulting in an individualized form of assistance for the student. All 3 forms of accommodation serve slightly different purposes, but all are uniquely responsive to the needs of the student while adhering to a common goal of maximizing the student-athlete's potential.

Temporary accommodations are broad in scope and can include adjusted assignment due dates, extended time for homework, longer testing periods, excused absence from school, assistance with reading tests, or physical modifications that ease the discomfort caused by certain environmental features like light and noise.[5] The primary purpose of these temporary measures is to provide an opportunity for recovery and symptom relief. Temporary accommodations allow for proper implementation of cognitive rest while salvaging the student's ability to participate in some or all parts of the formal school day. Temporary accommodations should be available to the student-athlete immediately following a concussion. This will avoid unnecessary academic complications and significant academic performance degradation. The process of establishing accommodations also facilitates understanding by school personnel about SRC and its potential impact on performance. At first, any adjustments to the normal academic routine should be made with and through the teachers who have daily responsibility for the student. Best practices would suggest that each school identify a point person to facilitate communication with the teachers.[4] If adjustments are anticipated to be needed longer than 3 to 5 weeks, then the informal adjustments negotiated with individual teachers may be formalized. This is implemented through a 504 plan, which references the section of the Rehabilitation Act that provides accommodation for those with medical need. To qualify for a 504 plan, an individual must display, through medical evaluation, that he or she has a physical or mental impairment that limits one or more major life activities.[4] A summary of this information can be found in Table 38-1.

Table 38-1			
Accommodation Types and Implementation Time Frames			
Type of Accommodation	**Definition**	**Time Frame**	**Implementation Mechanism**
Academic adjustment	Nonformalized changes in environment	3 to 5 weeks	Informal negotiation with teachers and academic administrators
Academic accommodation	Longer academic accommodation needs (ie, alternative arrangements for standardized testing)	5 weeks to 4 months	504 plan
Academic modification	More prolonged changes necessary (special education)	>4 to 6 months	Individualized Education Plan (IEP)

If school accommodations are necessary for longer than 4 to 6 months, accommodations available under the "special education" umbrella may be required and can only be granted through the implementation of an individualized education plan (IEP). An IEP is designed for people enrolled in public school education to receive special education. An IEP brings a collaboration of the school personnel and physicians together to best improve educational opportunities for individuals.[6] IEPs are available for individuals aged 3 to 21 years and require a medically documented disability in order to begin proper paperwork. IEPs and 504 plans are permanent documentation in the school system that allows for implementation of any necessary academic changes to make the student-athlete comfortable and academically successful. Both IEPs and 504 plans are re-evaluated, and changes can be made as necessary.

Despite the fact that these strategies for student reintegration into the classroom following an SRC exist, the frequent experience of students and their families attempting to take advantage of them is one of frustration. Although this situation is easing somewhat because of the significant public attention given to the topic of concussion, few schools have organized and coordinated their resources in a way that makes classroom adjustment a simple process for affected families. In these cases, parents are on their own to try to establish a point of contact within the school that can help facilitate the required adjustments. In these situations, athletic trainers can play an important role in bridging the gap between family and school and can help educate teachers and academic administrators about the needs of concussed students. Athletic trainers may also initiate an effort within the school to identify and develop a proper concussion-management team to implement necessary accommodations and to be consulted by families who require assistance in the wake of an SRC. Team physicians can also play a role by acknowledging the educational needs of their patients. They can educate parents and patients themselves about return-to-learn strategies and resources available to them. Like athletic trainers, team physicians can effectively initiate an effort to implement school-based solutions for the needs of their patients. Team physicians should also function on multidisciplinary resource teams composed of teachers, school counselors, and other personnel who can assist students in their reentry into the classroom.

References

1. Mealings M, Douglas J. 'School's a big part of your life...': adolescent perspectives of their school participation following traumatic brain injury. *Brain Impairment.* 2010;11:1-16.
2. McCrory P, McCrory P, Meeuwisse WH, et al. Consensus statement on concussion in sport: the 4th International Conference on Concussion in Sport held in Zurich, November 2012. *Br J Sports Med.* 2013;47:250-258.
3. Pope A, Tarlov A. A model for disability and disability prevention. In: A Pope, A Tarlov, eds. *Disability in America: Toward a National Agenda for Prevention.* Washington, DC: National Academy Press; 1991:76-108.
4. Halstead ME, McAvoy K, Devore CD, et al. Returning to learning following a concussion. *Pediatrics.* 2013;132:948-957.
5. McGrath N. Supporting the student-athlete's return to the classroom after a sport-related concussion. *J Athl Train.* 2010;45:492-498.
6. Piebes SK, Gourley M, Valovich McLeod TC. Caring for student-athletes following a concussion. *J Sch Nurs.* 2009;25:270-281.

HOW ARE EDUCATIONAL ACCOMMODATIONS DETERMINED, AND WHO SHOULD BE PART OF THE DECISION-MAKING PROCESS?

Richelle M. Williams, MS, ATC and
Tamara C. Valovich McLeod, PhD, ATC, FNATA

Concussion-management policies typically suggest both physical and cognitive rest as the key to concussion management. As stated in previous chapters, cognitive rest is the reduction in brain-stimulating mental activities.[1,2] These activities can include video games, television, reading, and schoolwork. In some cases, patients have difficulty with some or all aspects of academic activities, and it is necessary to provide academic accommodations. Academic accommodations may include temporary academic adjustments or more formal accommodations such as a 504 plan or Individualized Education Plan. The determination of academic accommodations should be made on a case-by-case basis with the input from an interdisciplinary team (Table 39-1).[3,4]

In order to facilitate educational accommodations, a team of school, family, and medical personnel should be involved. An athletic trainer, if available, a school nurse, academic personnel (principal, counselor, teachers), a physician, parents, and the student-athlete should be a part of the educational accommodation team. Prior

Valovich McLeod TC, ed. *Quick Questions in Sport-Related Concussion: Expert Advice in Sports Medicine* (pp 199-203).
© 2015 Taylor & Francis Group.

Table 39-1

Roles of Concussion Team Members for Implementing Educational Accommodations

Team	Team Members	Roles
Family	Patient, parents, guardians, relatives, peers, teammates, family friends	Impose rest Monitor and track symptoms at home, including emotional and sleep-related symptoms daily Communicate with school teams
Medical	Primary care provider, team physician, emergency department, concussion specialist, neuropsychologist, other medical referrals	Rule out more serious injury Evaluate patient periodically Coordinate information from other teams Encourage physical and cognitive rest
School: academic	School nurse, school counselor, teachers, school psychologist, social worker, school administrator, school physician, school occupational or physical therapist	Reduce cognitive load Meet with patient to create academic adjustments Watch, monitor, and track academic and emotional issues
School: physical activity	Athletic trainer, school nurse, coach, physical education teacher, school physician, playground supervisor	Watch, monitor, and track physical symptoms Athletic trainer should do daily follow-up examinations Ensure no physical activity

Adapted from McAvoy K. REAP the Benefits of Good Concussion Management. Rocky Mountain Hospital for Children. Published October 2013. © 2013 HCA-HealthONE LLC.

to the need for any accommodations for a concussed patient, the school should establish a concussion plan that includes the role of all personnel, evaluation schedule, and communication plan. All personnel should review and update this plan annually. Figure 39-1 depicts areas that should be included in the concussion plan.

If a student-athlete sustains a concussion, the coach, athletic trainer, or school nurse should notify the parents immediately. Communication should then be provided to the other concussion team members. This immediate communication can help facilitate implementation of temporary accommodations for the following day, should they be needed. In some instances, the severity of symptoms may result

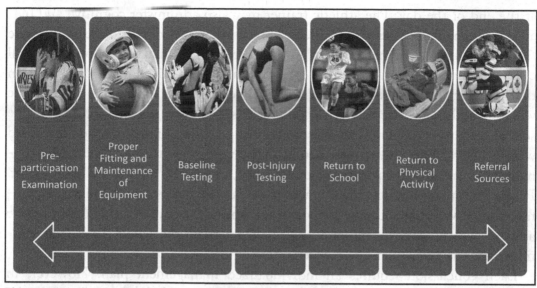

Figure 39-1. Concussion plan components.

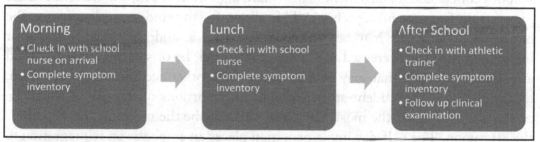

Figure 39-2. Daily follow-up at school.

in an excused absence from school in the acute period after injury[5]; however, one goal should be to return the student-athlete to a regular school day as soon as it is feasible.[6] The choice of academic accommodations should be made based on the patient's specific symptoms. For example, patients with light sensitivity may benefit from being allowed to wear sunglasses in the classroom, and patients with visual or vestibular problems should be encouraged to refrain from computer use.

In the days after the concussion, the team should implement the plan to enhance recovery for the student-athlete and ease him or her back into the educational setting. The needs and expectations of the patient can be addressed in a team manner and help to make the recovery time easier (Figure 39-2). The school nurse can evaluate the student first thing in the morning and monitor him or her throughout the school day. The student-athlete should understand that if symptoms increase or a rest break is needed, the school nurse is available to assist. The athletic trainer should be doing regular follow-up assessments and can assist in determining whether classroom activity provoked any symptoms through a symptom evaluation at the end of the day. The athletic trainer may also administer cognitive and balance assessments, the results of which can be used by the concussion team to revise the temporary accommodations plan. The treating primary care provider will evaluate the student-athlete periodically and can communicate with the school on the need for any changes to the educational accommodation plan and determine whether additional referrals are necessary based on the patient's progress. The school academic personnel can assist in ensuring all accommodations are discussed with teachers. This will ensure there is understanding of the need for the accommodations and that the patient is not punished for missing a test or an assignment. Parent and student-athlete involvement is vital to the success of educational accommodations. Without adequate support from family, the student-athlete may not be able to speak out when symptoms progress throughout the school day. Open communication is a key to ensure recovery.

Each concussion requires an individualized management plan. However, in general, the following recommendations should be considered for inclusion in the school's concussion management plan. Following a concussion, the student-athlete may refrain from attending school.[5] This allows for the student-athlete to rest the brain when he or she may be symptomatic. Once a student-athlete feels his or her symptoms have decreased to a manageable level, he or she can try a modified attendance schedule that may or may not include other accommodations. Often, this means that the student-athlete attends only portions of the day in which he or she is able to focus the most. For some, this may be the morning and for others the afternoon. The half-day implementation places an emphasis on reintegration to the classroom but allows the student-athlete to be in control of the workload. After symptoms have decreased in severity and quantity, a student-athlete may return to school for a full day but have accommodations in place. The specific accommodations will vary by patient but may include the student-athlete being allowed to excuse him- or herself to a quiet room if symptoms are triggered, having a reduced workload, or even wearing sunglasses in class. Similar to the progression used to return to physical activity, a classroom reintegration progression, sometimes termed *return-to-learn*,[6] should be used to slowly work up to school attendance for a full day, followed by the reduction of accommodations, as the student-athlete recovers. In the final few stages of recovery, the student-athlete would be able to attend a full school day without accommodations and then begin to reintegrate into after-school activities, with the eventual return to sports or recreational activities.

Although most concussions will resolve with the use of physical and cognitive rest and some temporary academic accommodations, there will be patients who have a more complicated recovery that may include prolonged symptoms. In these cases, additional referral sources, including neurologists or neuropsychologists, may be brought in as part of the concussion-management team. Should academic accommodations need to be implemented over a longer period of time, the concussion team may identify a 504 plan as a better way to provide accommodations. In this case, additional individuals may join the concussion team to ensure all 504 policies are being followed and appropriate assessments of the student are completed. As with other areas of concussion management, the use of educational accommodations is a dynamic process that will include a variety of individuals, depending on the stage of recovery and clinical presentation of the student-athlete. Having an appropriate concussion team in place to oversee academic accommodations is essential in helping the student-athlete recover from his or her concussion successfully and safely.

References

1. Valovich McLeod TC, Gioia GA. Cognitive rest: the often neglected aspect of concussion management. *Athlet Ther Today.* 2010;15(2):1-3.
2. Moser RS, Glatts C, Schatz P. Efficacy of immediate and delayed cognitive and physical rest for treatment of sports-related concussion. *J Pediatr.* 2012;161(5):922-926 .
3. Rocky Mountain Youth Sports Medicine Institute Center for Concussion. REAP Guidelines. http://issuu.com/healthone/docs/reap_oct21. Accessed February 27, 2014.
4. Piebes SK, Gourley M, Valovich McLeod TC. Caring for student-athletes following a concussion. *J Sch Nurs.* 2009;25(4):270-281.
5. McGrath N. Supporting the student-athlete's return to the classroom after a sport-related concussion. *J Athl Train.* 2010;45(5):492-498.
6. Halstead ME, McAvoy K, Devore CD, Carl R, Lee M, Logan K. Returning to learning following a concussion. *Pediatrics.* 2013;132(5):948-957.

FINANCIAL DISCLOSURES

Dr. Matthew Anastasi has no financial or proprietary interest in the materials presented herein.

Ms. Erica L. Beidler has no financial or proprietary interest in the materials presented herein.

Dr. Steven P. Broglio has no financial or proprietary interest in the materials presented herein.

Dr. Javier Cárdenas is an Unaffiliated Neurotrauma Consultant for and on the Head, Neck & Spine Committee for the National Football League.

Dr. Meeryo C. Choe has no financial or proprietary interest in the materials presented herein.

Dr. Michael W. Collins is co-developer and board member of ImPACT Applications, Inc.

Dr. Tracey Covassin has no financial or proprietary interest in the materials presented herein.

Ms. Laura Decoster has no financial or proprietary interest in the materials presented herein.

Dr. R.J. Elbin has no financial or proprietary interest in the materials presented herein.

Dr. Steven Erickson has no financial or proprietary interest in the materials presented herein.

205

Ms. Sheri Fedor has no financial or proprietary interest in the materials presented herein.

Dr. Christopher C. Giza has no financial or proprietary interest in the materials presented herein.

Dr. Anthony P. Kontos has no financial or proprietary interest in the materials presented herein.

Dr. Christina B. Kunec has no financial or proprietary interest in the materials presented herein.

Ms. Ashley C. Littleton has no financial or proprietary interest in the materials presented herein.

Dr. Scott C. Livingston has no financial or proprietary interest in the materials presented herein.

Mr. Robert C. Lynall has no financial or proprietary interest in the materials presented herein.

Mr. Douglas Martini has no financial or proprietary interest in the materials presented herein.

Ms. Shelly Massingale has no financial or proprietary interest in the materials presented herein.

Dr. Roger McCoy has no financial or proprietary interest in the materials presented herein.

Mr. Ian A. McLeod has no financial or proprietary interest in the materials presented herein.

Dr. Jason P. Mihalik has no financial or proprietary interest in the materials presented herein.

Ms. Valerie Needham has no financial or proprietary interest in the materials presented herein.

Dr. John T. Parsons has no financial or proprietary interest in the materials presented herein.

Dr. Danielle M.E. Ransom has no financial or proprietary interest in the materials presented herein.

Dr. Johna K. Register-Mihalik has no financial or proprietary interest in the materials presented herein.

Dr. Julianne D. Schmidt has no financial or proprietary interest in the materials presented herein.

Ms. Lindsey Shepherd has no financial or proprietary interest in the materials presented herein.

Dr. Amaal J. Starling has no financial or proprietary interest in the materials presented herein.

Dr. Tamara C. Valovich McLeod has no financial or proprietary interest in the materials presented herein.

Dr. Christopher G. Vaughan has no financial or proprietary interest in the materials presented herein.

Ms. Jessica Wallace has no financial or proprietary interest in the materials presented herein.

Ms. Michelle L. Weber has no financial or proprietary interest in the materials presented herein.

Ms. Richelle M. Williams has no financial or proprietary interest in the materials presented herein.

Dr. Kristina Wilson has no financial or proprietary interest in the materials presented herein.

Mr. Max Zeiger has no financial or proprietary interest in the materials presented herein.

INDEX

Printed in the United States
by Baker & Taylor Publisher Services